SEP 1 PAID

D1260979

FORTRAN
PROGRAMMING

BY THE SAME AUTHOR:

Introductory Computer Programming, 1966

FORTRAN PROGRAMMING

Fredric Stuart

Department of Business Statistics
Hofstra University

JOHN WILEY & SONS, INC.

New York · London · Sydney · Toronto

Photographs courtesy of Burroughs Corporation, Control Data Corporation, Digital Equipment Corporation, Electronic Associates, Inc., General Electric Company, International Business Machines Corporation, International Computers and Tabulators, Ltd., National Cash Register Company, Radio Corporation of America, Raytheon Company, Scientific Data Systems, and Systems Engineering Laboratories, Inc.

Copyright © 1969 by Fredric Stuart

All rights reserved. No part of this book may be reproduced by any means, nor transmitted, nor translated into a machine language without the written permission of the publisher.

10 9 8 7 6 5 4 3 2

Library of Congress Catalog Card Number: 68–30922

SBN 471 83477 7

Printed in the United States of America

To Freda

PREFACE

This book is intended as both textbook and reference manual for the FORTRAN computer programming language. It has been designed for use with any computer for which FORTRAN is available. This intercomputer applicability is implemented by twenty-five reference tables appearing throughout the text, which index specific FORTRAN statements for 152 computer models, by text explanations of alternative statement forms, and by a summary comparison table in Appendix B.

When the boss asks "Can you use our computer?" the employee should *not* respond:

	(*a*)	only if you provide a programmer
or	(*b*)	only if it is an IBM 1620, Model II
or	(*c*)	only if it uses the ZIPPY-QUIK language
or	(*d*)	only if it uses FORTRAN II
or	(*e*)	only if it uses FORTRAN IV

Our central purpose is to provide the correct response,

(*f*) yes (unless it is a rather small computer).

Though the "computer revolution" is still in its early stages, we have already reached a point at which almost all college students, many high school students, and very large numbers of practicing professional and business people have one or more computers available for their use. But most of these people have not yet taken advantage of this availability.

In many cases they assume that direct usage is the province of computer *experts*—that somebody called a "programmer" must be consulted, for translation of any problem to computer terms (answer *a*). In other instances, a little exposure to machine language or assembler language programming has left them with the ability to program only *one* computer model, which inevitably is out of style by now (answer *b*). Some have learned shortcut programming languages which are implemented for very few computers (answer *c*). Others (answers *d* and *e*) have been set on the right track by learning FORTRAN, but are prevented from a "Yes" response by the apparent coexistence of dozens of *dialects* of the FORTRAN language. Since they have learned only one such dialect, they are uncertain as to applicability to the computer that now confronts them.

There are at present more than 200 computer models in use. Nearly 80 per cent of them are provided with FORTRAN *compiler* programs, which enable the computer to translate from FORTRAN (which uses English and basic arithmetic notation) to its own "machine language." Although machine languages are highly individual for each computer, the FORTRAN language is really quite uniform. It was designed as a machine-independent language suitable for all computers and has been widely accepted as such by manufacturers.

The evolution from "FORTRAN" to "FORTRAN II" to "FORTRAN IV" (FORTRAN III, like the P-39 fighter plane, apparently never existed), which is still continuing, has *enlarged* the language, but has not produced any real obstacle to treatment of all the versions as a *single* FORTRAN language.

The computer-to-computer FORTRAN differences that do exist cannot really be classified by describing a given compiler as "FORTRAN II" or "FORTRAN IV." Our comparison tables indicate that, although individual statement differences are each minor and easily adjusted for, there are actually more than seventy "different" compilers, created by various *combinations* of the differences. For this reason, several problems—shifting of FORTRAN programs from one computer to another, writing programs in FORTRAN language that will be acceptable to a large number of (or some specific collection of) computers, and making computer acquisition and rental decisions with regard to FORTRAN capabilities—cannot be solved by two-word classification of compilers, but may be solved by use of the reference materials herein.

Although the compiler-comparison tables have been prepared by careful study of computer manufacturers' FORTRAN Reference Manuals, the *textbook* that surrounds the tables departs radically from the usual order of presentation to be found in such manuals, and indeed in many textbooks. Instead of introducing whole *categories* of FORTRAN statements by listing all members of a class at once, the text introduces the student to the simpler forms of each statement type; after he has practiced with these, he is presented with additional (frequently more elegant) statements of each type. Thus the *control* statement is represented in Chapter 2 only by the unconditional GO TO statement; the Arithmetic IF statement is not added until Chapter 4, the DO statement appears in Chapter 5, conditional GO TO statements and Logical IF statements are deferred until Chapter 8, and CALL and RETURN statements until Chapter 9. The same gradual introduction is followed for *arithmetic* statements, *input/output* statements, *specification* statements, and *variable types*.

One very important deferment is the placement of detailed discussion of FORMAT in Chapter 6. For the many sample programs in the text, and for exercise programs written by the student, earlier chapters provide a *"standard"* FORMAT statement, which is used for both input and output. I have found in my own teaching that students faced with learning basic computation techniques and input/output arrangements simultaneously become hopelessly mired down in the complexities of the latter, at a time when they should be convincing themselves that instructing the computer in FORTRAN is easy.

Since FORTRAN cannot be learned by merely reading about it, 120 practice exercises are provided; most of them outline problems, drawn from a variety of disciplines, for which complete (usually short) FORTRAN programs may be written. The subject areas represented in the exercises include simple arithmetic, elementary logic, statistics, business data processing, mathematics, engineering, chemistry, geology, physics, linguistics, and the behavioral sciences. Each problem, however, is sufficiently self-contained (e.g., necessary computation formulas are provided) to permit programming by students not conversant with the originating discipline.

The student is encouraged to compile and execute on the computer as many of the exercise programs as he can, as an indispensable aid to the learning process. To facilitate debugging and testing of student programs, correct *output* for each exercise problem appears in Appendix A. Exercise programs requiring *data* have all been tested on a *standard data set*, consisting of twenty punched cards, which is listed at the beginning of Appendix A.

All textbook authors share some obvious motivations. Aside from the baser economic and political ones, we all hope to *teach* somebody something. In this work, that purpose should be served by the careful ordering of subject matter from easy to difficult, by the inclusion of large numbers of example programs, and by the provision of exercises (with sample output) drawn from a large variety of disciplines.

Our hopes for the compiler-comparison tables, however, are somewhat broader. For the beginning student, these tables have limited usefulness, since he is really concerned with only one line of each—the line corresponding to the computer he is learning with. In addition to solving the specific program-shifting problems listed earlier, the tables should demonstrate convincingly that there *is* a "universal" computer programming language—and thereby advance the *cause* of FORTRAN.

I happen to believe that, since the computer is useful to millions of people, millions of people should learn to program it. And the splintering of the field into noncompatible languages stands as a serious obstacle to this learning process. It may be too late for all nations to agree on Esperanto—but there is still time for all computer users to agree on FORTRAN.[1]

A number of linguists, fluent in both FORTRAN and their own professional jargons, have been of great help in reading the manuscript, offering many constructive suggestions which have been incorporated, and providing exercise problems drawn from their own fields. My thanks to Dr. Sheldon Blackman, Professor Benjamin F. Chi, William S. Dorn, Dr. Kenneth M. Goldstein, Dr. George W. Logemann, Professor Donald G. McBrien, Professor Daniel F. Merriam, Philip G. Meynen, Thomas A. Murrell, Professor Warren Seider. Any errors, of course, are attributable neither to them *nor* to me. We blame various computers, which shall be nameless.

Glen Head, New York   FREDRIC STUART
July, 1968

---

[1] As a general-purpose language. I do not deny the usefulness of some specialized languages for special purposes, nor the possibility of eventual replacement of FORTRAN by a *better* general-purpose language. What I am arguing for is as much language standardization as possible, to assure intercomputer shiftability of programs and users.

CONTENTS

INDEX
OF FORTRAN
COMPILERS

Tables 1 to 25 in the text, and a summary table in Appendix B, list availability and form of specific FORTRAN statements for 78 compilers provided for a total of 152 computer models. The compilers, applicable computer models, and manufacturers are listed below, with compiler reference numbers which are used in the tables. The 79th line of each table ("USAS") shows FORTRAN IV standards set by the U.S.A. Standards Institute.

Compiler Reference Number	Computer Models	Number of Models	Manufacturer
1	Adage AMBILOG 200	1	Adage, Incorporated
	ADVANCE (*see* EMR)		
2	ARGUS 400, 500	2	Ferranti Electric, Inc.
3	Burroughs B2500, B3500	2	Burroughs Corporation
4	Burroughs B5500	1	Burroughs Corporation
5	Burroughs B6500, B7500, B8500	3	Burroughs Corporation
6	Collins C-8500	1	Collins Radio Company
7	Control Data 160	1	Control Data Corporation
8	Control Data 160A	1	Control Data Corporation
9	Control Data 1604, 1604A	2	Control Data Corporation
10	Control Data 1700	1	Control Data Corporation
11	Control Data 3100, 3150, 3200, 3300, 3500	5	Control Data Corporation
12	Control Data 3100, 3200 (Basic)		Control Data Corporation
13	Control Data 3400, 3600, 3800 (including SUMMIT FORTRAN)	3	Control Data Corporation
14	Control Data 6400, 6500, 6600, 7600 (CHIPPEWA FORTRAN)	4	Control Data Corporation
15	Control Data 6400, 6500, 6600, 7600 (EXTENDED FORTRAN)		Control Data Corporation
16	Control Data G-20 (FORTRAN II)	1	Control Data Corporation

Compiler Reference Number	Computer Models	Number of Models	Manufacturer
17	Control Data G-20 (FORTRAN M)		Control Data Corporation
18	Data Machines 620, 620I	2	Data Machines, Incorporated
	DDP (*see* Honeywell DDP)		
19	DIGIAC 3080	1	Digital Electronics, Inc.
20	Digital Equipment PDP-8	1	Digital Equipment Corporation
21	Digital Equipment PDP-9	1	Digital Equipment Corporation
22	Digital Equipment PDP-10	1	Digital Equipment Corporation
23	EAI 640	1	Electronic Associates, Inc.
24	EAI 8400	1	Electronic Associates, Inc.
25	Elliott 903	1	Elliott Automation Group
26	Elliott 4120, 4130	2	Elliott Automation Group
27	EMR ADVANCE 6020, 6040, 6050, 6070	4	Electro-Mechanical Research Inc.
	Ferranti (*see* ARGUS)		
28	English Electric 4-30	1	English Electric Computers, Ltd.
29	English Electric 4-50	1	English Electric Computers, Ltd.
30	English Electric KDF-9	1	English Electric Computers, Ltd.
	GEC 90/25, 90/30, 90/300 (*see* Scientific Data SDS 925, 930, 9300)		
	GEC S.2, S.7 (*see* Scientific Data SIGMA 2, SIGMA 7)		
31	General Electric 205, 215, 225, 235 (card)	4	General Electric Company
32	General Electric 205, 215, 225, 235 (tape)		General Electric Company
33	General Electric 412, 415, 425, 435	4	General Electric Company
34	General Electric 625, 635, 645	3	General Electric Company
35	General Electric GE/PAC 4020, 4040, 4050I, 4050II, 4060	5	General Electric Company
36	General Electric Time-Sharing		General Electric Company
37	Honeywell 200/120, /200, /1200, /2200, /4200, /8200	6	Honeywell; Electronic Data Processing Division
38	Honeywell DDP-24, -124, -224, -416, -516	5	Honeywell; Computer Control Division
39	Hughes H-330, H-3324	2	Hughes Aircraft Company
40	IBM 360 (OS, DOS, TOS, BPS)		International Business Machines Corporation

(*continued*)

Compiler Reference Number	Computer Models	Number of Models	Manufacturer
41	IBM 360 (BPSC —"E" LEVEL)	7	International Business Machines Corporation
42	IBM 360-44PS ("G", "H" Levels)		International Business Machines Corporation
43	IBM 360 Time-Sharing (360-67)		International Business Machines Corporation
44	IBM 1130	1	International Business Machines Corporation
45	IBM 1401	1	International Business Machines Corporation
46	IBM 1410	1	International Business Machines Corporation
47	IBM 1401, 1440, 1460	2	International Business Machines Corporation
48	IBM 1620I, 1620II	2	International Business Machines Corporation
49	IBM 1800	1	International Business Machines Corporation
50	IBM 1410, 7010	1	International Business Machines Corporation
51	IBM 7040, 7044 (8K)	2	International Business Machines Corporation
52	IBM 7040, 7044 (16–32K)		International Business Machines Corporation
53	IBM 7070	1	International Business Machines Corporation
54	IBM 7080	1	International Business Machines Corporation
55	IBM 7090, 7094I, 7094II	3	International Business Machines Corporation
56	ICT 1901, 1902, 1903, 1904, 1905, 1906, 1907, 1909	8	International Computers & Tabulators, Ltd.
57	ICT ATLAS 2	1	International Computers & Tabulators, Ltd.
58	ICT ORION 2	1	International Computers & Tabulators, Ltd.
59	NCR 315, 315/100, 315/RMC 501, 315/RMC 502 (FORTRAN II)	4	National Cash Register Company
60	NCR 315, 315/100, 315/RMC 501, 315/RMC 502 (FORTRAN IV)		National Cash Register Company

Compiler Reference Number	Computer Models	Number of Models	Manufacturer
	PDP (*see* Digital Equipment)		
61	Philco 2000/210, /211, /212, /213	4	Philco Corporation
	PRODAC 250 (*see* Scientific Data SIGMA 2)		
62	Raytheon 250	1	Raytheon Company
63	Raytheon 520	1	Raytheon Company
64	RCA SPECTRA 70/15, /25, /35, /45, /46, /55	6	Radio Corporation of America
65	RCA 301	1	Radio Corporation of America
66	RCA 3301	1	Radio Corporation of America
67	Scientific Control 650, 655, 660/2, 660/5, 670/2	5	Scientific Control Corporation
68	Scientific Data SDS 910, 920, 925, 930, 940, 9300	6	Scientific Data Systems
69	Scientific Data SIGMA 2	1	Scientific Data Systems
70	Scientific Data SIGMA 5, SIGMA 7	2	Scientific Data Systems
71	SEL 810A, 810B	2	Systems Engineering Laboratories, Inc.
72	SEL 840A, 840MP	2	Systems Engineering Laboratories, Inc.
73	UNIVAC 418	1	Sperry Rand Corporation, UNIVAC Division
74	UNIVAC 490, 491, 492, 494	4	Sperry Rand Corporation, UNIVAC Division
75	UNIVAC 1050	1	Sperry Rand Corporation, UNIVAC Division
76	UNIVAC 1107	1	Sperry Rand Corporation, UNIVAC Division
77	UNIVAC 1108	1	Sperry Rand Corporation, UNIVAC Division
78	UNIVAC U-III	1	Sperry Rand Corporation, UNIVAC Division
	Westinghouse PRODAC 250 (*see* Scientific Data SIGMA 2)		
79	U.S.A. Standards Institute, Standards for FORTRAN IV		

TABLES

FORTRAN
PROGRAMMING

1 • INTRODUCTION

This book will teach you how to *use* electronic computers. The italics serve as warning that you are not embarked on a computer-appreciation course. There will be no discussion of the social and economic implications of computers, nor of the electronic basis of their performance. A competent computer user has no more need for detailed knowledge of circuits, gates, and registers than the adding-machine user has for knowledge of cams, gears and rollers.

You will discover, in fact, that the surest route to appreciation of what the computer is and does is the most direct one—learn to use it. This learning process is neither long nor difficult. You can start writing complete programs almost immediately; a few weeks of study will permit you to translate real problems from your own field of specialization, for direct action by the computer; a few months of practice should relieve you of dependence on that unsatisfactory middleman, the "programmer." This achievement of the most practical form of mastery over the computer will not make you a "computer expert"; but, in addition to permitting direct usage, it will certainly give you a precise idea of what computers can and cannot do.

People who do not learn to program the computer tend toward two opposite errors as to its capabilities. On the one hand, there is the notion that the computer is a fast combination adding machine/addressograph which is the exclusive property of the Accounting Department down the hall. It has been designed by a manufacturer with a specific set of rote jobs in mind, and only certain handpicked personnel trained by the manufacturer dare interfere with the superefficient accomplishment of these tasks.

At the other extreme, there is the notion that the computer "thinks" and that its introduction on the premises relieves the owners (or renters) of the troublesome tasks of (a) problem-solving and (b) decision-making. After some short period during which the computer is taught the fundamentals of the subject area, it may be left to itself to formulate questions, explore alternative answers, publish the results, and answer the telephone.

1

The truth, which obviously lies somewhere in between, begins with this statement: every problem that the computer "solves" is in principle solved by men, who write computer *programs*. A program is a step-by-step list of instructions that the computer is to follow. The computer will do nothing unless it has been directed explicitly to do it; and if a logical error is present in the instructions, it will blithely produce wrong answers with great speed and accuracy.

Early electronic computers (post-World War II) could be "programmed" (i.e., supplied with a fresh set of instructions) only by rewiring parts of circuits. A gradual evolution produced "written" programs, which could be transmitted to the computer in the same manner as numerical data (using punched cards, paper tape, magnetic tape). But such instructions were written in a simple digital-code *machine language*, which was limited to a short set of operations (add, divide, print, and so on) and which was different for each computer make and model. *Assembler* languages also were provided, which substitute mnemonic labels (e.g., A for *add*) for much of the digital content of machine languages, but otherwise share the principal machine language disadvantages: there is usually a one-to-one correspondence between assembler language and machine language statements, and each assembler language is usable only on the computer for which it is designed.

In the late 1950's the idea of intermediate ("problem-oriented, machine-independent") languages reached full development with FORTRAN, ALGOL, COBOL, and others. Programs in these languages are more readily written and read by programmers, but require translation to the computer's machine language before execution of the programmer's instructions. This translation can be accomplished *by* the computer, acting on a set of instructions that themselves constitute a stored machine language program (the *compiler* program).

FORTRAN, which stands for "formula translation," is a language written in short phrases (*statements*) that utilize ordinary English and basic algebraic notation. A FORTRAN compiler program (which translates from FORTRAN to machine language) is provided for nearly 80 per cent of all computer models currently in use (there are more than 200 models, produced by more than 30 manufacturers). Thus programs written in FORTRAN can be executed by the great majority of computers. Though FORTRAN versions for different computers vary in certain details, they are dialects of a common language.

Before we begin our examination of the FORTRAN language, we shall describe briefly the kinds of equipment required for transmission and storage of the programmer's instructions and data and for output of the computer's results.

Digital Computers

You will be programming a *digital*, as opposed to an *analog*, computer. The distinction is simply that between *counting* and *measurement*. A subway turnstile (with traffic counter) is an elementary form of digital computer, while a thermometer may be described as a rudimentary analog computer.

Whereas digital computers represent numerical quantities as actual sets of

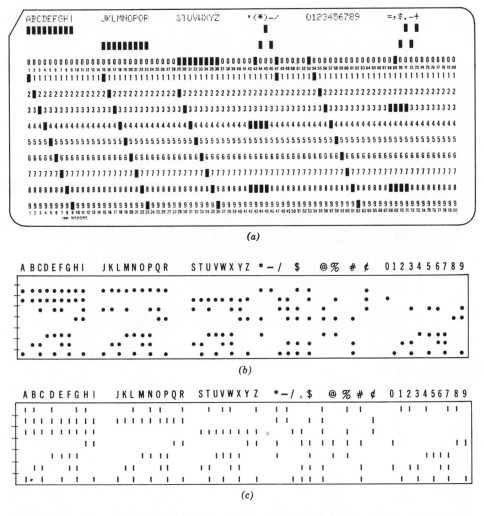

(a)

(b)

(c)

FIG. 1 (*a*) A punched-card alphabet. (*b*) A paper-tape alphabet. (*c*) A magnetic-tape alphabet.

digits, analog computers represent them as continuous amounts of some measurable physical entity (e.g., voltage). In terms of your own experience, you have used digital computation equipment when employing adding machines or desk calculators, and analog computation when employing a slide rule. So far as electronic computers are concerned, the digital type has become by far the most common, and it is for this type that FORTRAN is usually available.

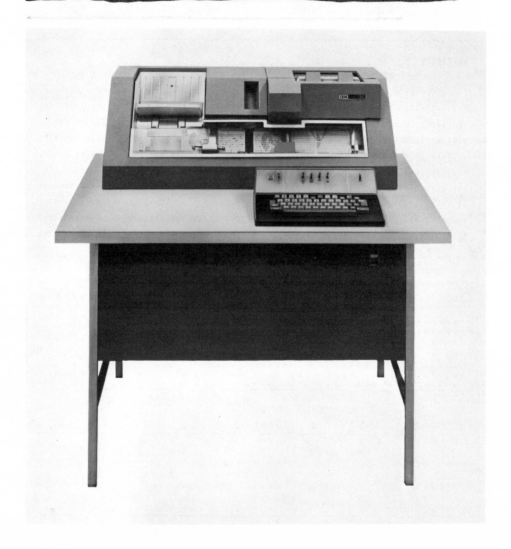

FIG. 2   IBM 029 keypunch machine.

Transmission to the Computer

With the exception of a few special-purpose computers that can "read" directly numeric and alphabetic characters written with special ink, the current generation of computers require translation to sets of holes in punched cards or paper tape, or electronic marks on magnetic tape. Commonly used alphabets for these input media, consisting of digits 1 through 9, letters A through Z, and selected special characters (plus sign, decimal point, etc.), appear in Fig. 1.

Careful study of these arrangements is *not* necessary, since the translation from written symbols is not the programmer's responsibility; it is accomplished by a typewriterlike device whose keyboard contains all characters that may be represented. Figure 2 shows a keypunch machine, used for punching cards.

Examples of input equipment required for entering cards or tape are shown in Fig. 3. A typical arrangement for cards consists of 80 wire brushes, which complete electrical contact with a metal plate when a card passing between brushes and plate contains a punched hole. The combination of brush number and precise timing of the contact defines the character that is to be passed into storage. For example, a single punch in the fourth row of the first column will result in a recording of the digit "4" in computer storage. All 80 columns are read simultaneously.

Punched cards are available as an input medium for most computer systems and are more convenient than tape for the transmission of short separate programs. Other input media available in various combinations include:

> paper tape
> magnetic tape
> typewriter or teletype
> magnetic character reader or optical scanner

Some of these will be discussed in connection with computer output. First, however, we should look at the provisions for storage of programs and data.

Computer Storage

The computer's main storage is contained in the *central processor* (see Fig. 4), which also serves as the control and computation unit (as opposed to input/output units). This area is known as the *primary* storage. It contains thousands of individual units ("bits"), each of which has two possible states—magnetized or unmagnetized, or magnetization in one of two directions. In conformance to our avoidance of electronic discussions, let us think of each "bit" as simply "on" or "off."

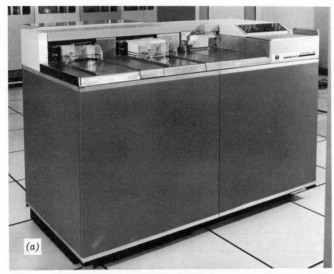

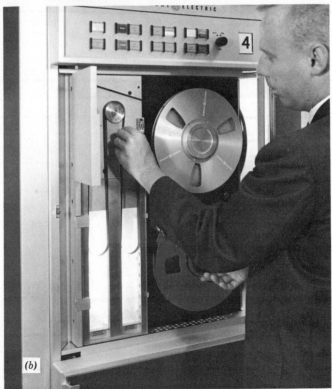

FIG. 3 (*a*) RCA Spectra 70/237 card reader. (*b*) General Electric MY-17 magnetic-tape handler.

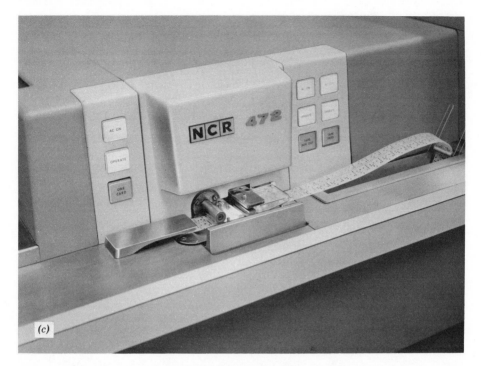

FIG. 3   (c) National Cash Register 472 paper-tape reader.

Primary storage is divided into groups of such bits, each group ("cell") designed to hold a numeric value. Two methods, both based on the binary number system, are used for the storage in each cell. In the more common straight binary system, the number 21 could be represented in a five-bit[1] cell:

x		x		x
16	8	4	2	1

STRAIGHT BINARY SYSTEM

In a "binary-coded decimal" system, the same number could be represented by two separate cells, each of which contained four bits for the purpose:

	8
	4
x	2
	1

	8
	4
	2
x	1

BINARY-CODED DECIMAL

---

[1] Individual numerical locations are generally larger than those shown here, to accommodate large numbers.

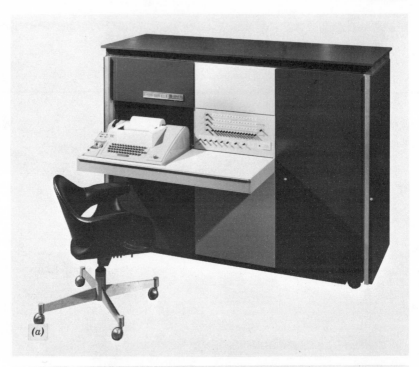

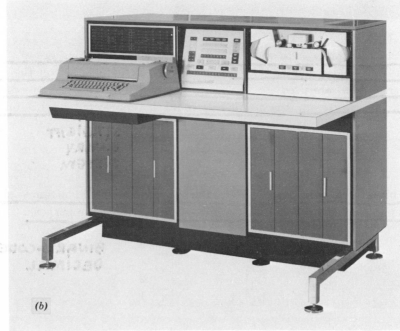

FIG. 4 Central processor and control console. (*a*) SEL 810A. (*b*) EAI 8400.

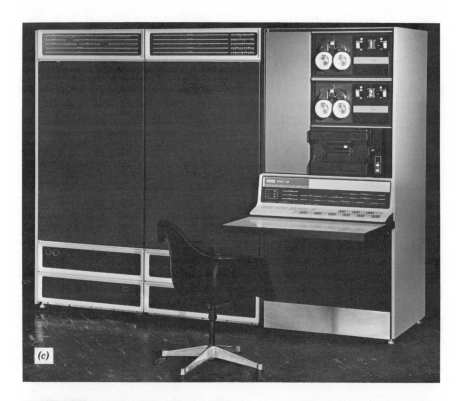

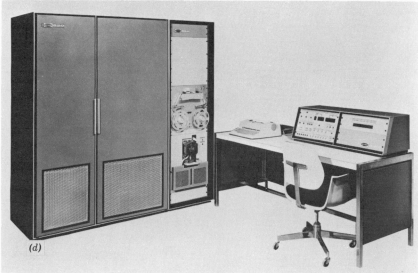

FIG. 4   (c) PDP-10. (d) Raytheon 520.

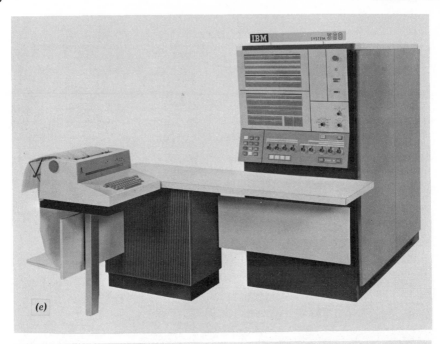

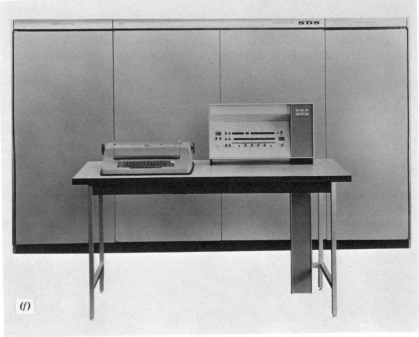

FIG. 4 (e) IBM 360. (f) SDS 930.

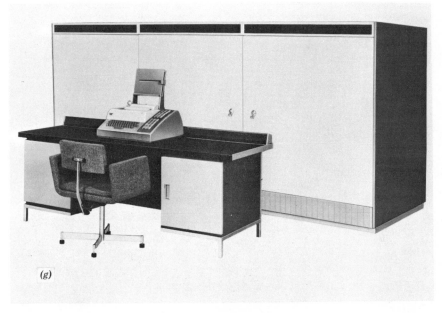

(g)

FIG. 4   (g) ICT 1904.

In either system, this "primary" storage is reached by *random access*. That is, any part of the storage can be reached without physically traveling through parts ahead of it. Thus any cell may be reached in the same total *access time* as any other. Many systems are provided with additional *secondary* storage—magnetic disk, tape, drum, and so on—which is "on-line" (i.e., is accessible from the computer's primary storage and its input/output equipment),[2] but may not provide random access.

Computer Output

Most computer systems have at least two on-line output devices, and some have multiple alternatives, including

typewriter or teletype	magnetic tape
on-line printer	magnetic disk or drum
plotter	video display
punched cards	verbal output
paper tape	

---

[2] "On-line" also signifies that the equipment is under direct control of the computer and therefore, of course, of the programmer.

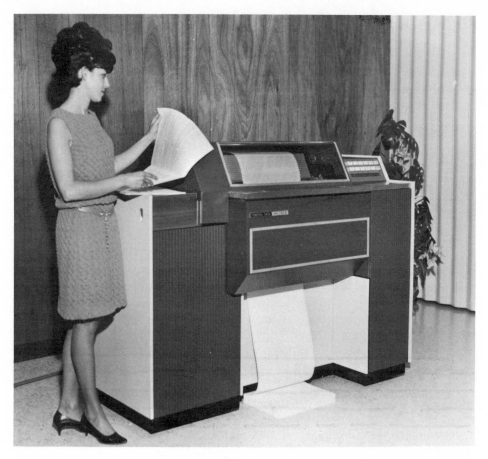

FIG. 5 Control Data line printer.

A typewriter, which usually stands on the computer console (see Fig. 4), is the slowest of these output devices, since it reproduces one character at a time, just as a typist would. On-line printers, on the other hand, reproduce in units of complete lines, usually 120 characters wide. One is shown in Fig. 5.

Output produced on punched cards, paper tape, or magnetic tape is in convenient form for further use as input data, but must be "listed" by using a piece of off-line equipment, if actual printed output is required. Most computers are "output-bound," that is, they can compute much more quickly than they can output results. Since on-line printing is frequently the computer's slowest activity, production of output on tape, and subsequent off-line conversion to print by specialized equipment, is a common practice.

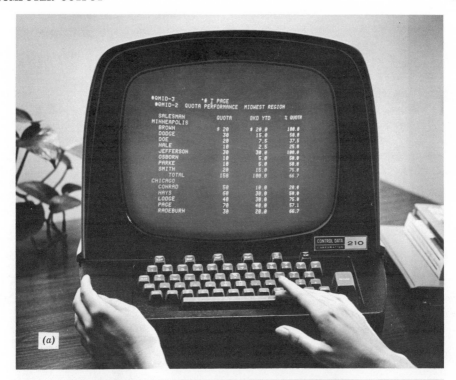

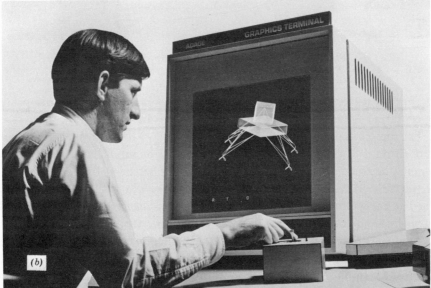

FIG. 6 (a) Control Data 210 video terminal. (b) Adage graphics terminal.

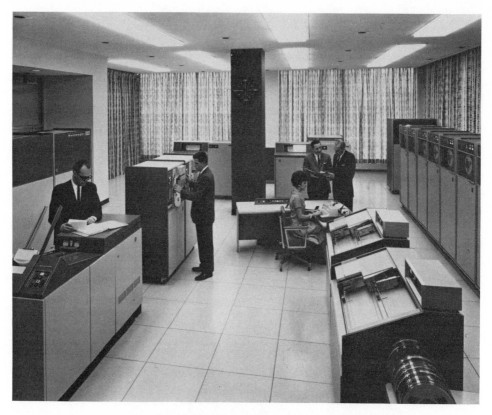

FIG. 7   The Burroughs B5500 computer system.

The plotter is a specialized piece of equipment that produces graphic representation (generally, line drawings) of values in storage.

The direction of output to an on-line, out-of-core location such as magnetic disk or drum is also for the purpose of further use as input data. An important difference between this kind of storage and that afforded by cards or tape is that the disk or drum provides access that is very nearly *random* (as we have defined it earlier for core storage), rather than *sequential*. One cannot read a number from the middle of a tape without winding through half the reel.

"Video display" (see Fig. 6) refers to cathode ray scopes, which are efficient when no permanent record of output is required, especially when the output is of interest to an audience. They are appropriate, for example, for information retrieval systems (e.g., at airlines, banks). Another advantage, which has made the device popular with some scientists, is instant *graphic* display of results.

Verbal output, not yet very common, is usually accomplished by the use of collections of prerecorded sounds, from among which the computer selects (as directed by the programmer, of course). Thus the computer may be made to "speak" the answers, "play" music, or engage in other deceptively creative enterprise.

Figure 7 shows a complete system, incorporating several input/output alternatives.

For Review

program
machine language
assembler language
compiler program
FORTRAN
digital computer
analog computer
special character
keypunch
paper tape
magnetic tape
central processor
primary storage
bit
cell
straight binary system
binary-coded decimal system
random access
access time
on-line
secondary storage
plotter
magnetic disk
sequential access
listing

2 • INTRODUCTION TO FORTRAN

Let us examine a complete FORTRAN program, for a rather trivial problem. We shall have the computer compute and print total pay for a worker who completes 38 hours of work, at a wage rate of $3.17 per hour:

```
C        TOTAL PAY
         PAY = 38.0 * 3.17
         WRITE (3,100) PAY
100      FORMAT (5F15.5)
         END
```

The programmer should use a standard FORTRAN coding form (Fig. 8), to facilitate the keypunching process. Note that the form shown provides 80 columns, which correspond to the standard 80-column punched card, and that each FORTRAN statement occupies a separate line.

FORTRAN statements begin in column 7, while statement *numbers* (if used) appear in the first five columns. A statement cannot extend beyond column 72. The last eight columns may be used, however, for nonstatement purposes (e.g., sequence numbers or other identification codes), since they are ignored by the compiler program.

Each line will be keypunched as a separate card (Fig. 9), for the computer analyzes each card as an individual FORTRAN statement. An exception to this rule permits the programmer to *continue* long statements on successive cards, indicating the continuation by placement of a nonzero digit in column 6 of each continuation card, a column otherwise left blank. Cards with blank or zero in column 6 will be interpreted as new statements, while cards containing any other character in column 6 are interpreted as continuation lines. Table 1 shows the statement-continuation rule for various FORTRAN compilers. (This is the first of 25 such reference tables. To use the table, first look up the appropriate compiler reference number for your computer in the compiler index table that follows the Contents.)

Blank columns are usually ignored (some exceptions are discussed in

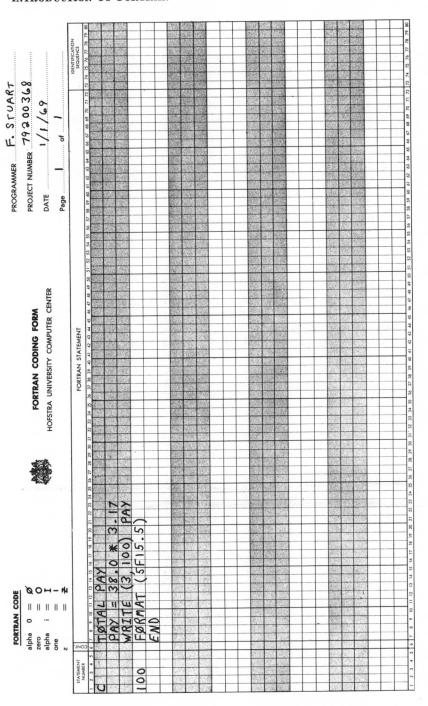

FIG. 8 The sample program as it appears on FORTRAN coding paper. You should adopt the conventional manner illustrated for writing the letter Ø, to distinguish it from the number 0. Similarly, I is by convention alphabetic and 1 is numeric (note that our type face in sample programs differs here; do not imitate it). Finally, the letter Z is written with a horizontal intersecting line, to avoid confusion with numeric 2.

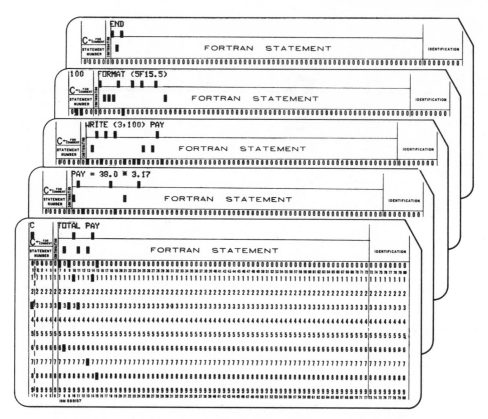

FIG. 9 The sample programs as it appears on punched cards.

Chapter 6) and may be used to improve legibility. That is, statements may be "stretched" horizontally by separation of words and symbols.

When the keypunch operator has completed the transfer from coding form to card deck (five cards for our sample program), the program is ready for transmission to the computer.

But—is the computer ready to receive a FORTRAN program? We have indicated earlier that each computer can interpret directly only its distinctive "machine language." Preparation for the FORTRAN program therefore requires insertion of the compiler program (in machine language form), which contains instructions on translating from FORTRAN to machine language. This program may itself be available as a deck of punched cards (or a reel of tape), which are entered ahead of the FORTRAN program cards. As an alternative, in systems provided with sufficient secondary storage capacity, the compiler

TABLE 1

FORTRAN Statement Continuation

	Not Permitted	Maximum Total Lines	Unlimited	Number Not Stated	Other
1[a]		6			
2			✓		
3			✓		
4					Maximum 700 characters
5			✓		
6		9			
7			✓		
8				✓	
9					Maximum 598 operators, delimiters, and identifiers
10		6			Maximum 202 operators, delimiters, and identifiers
11					$2n + m \leq 500$; n = identifiers, m = symbols and constants
12				✓	
13					Maximum 598 operators, delimiters, and identifiers
14		20			
15		20			
16		10			
17		10			
18			✓		
19	✓				
20					Maximum 128 characters
21			✓		
22		20			
23				✓	
24				✓	
25					Paper tape only; maximum 120 characters
26			✓		
27			✓		

[a] Compiler number.

TABLE 1 (*continued*)

	Not Permitted	Maximum Total Lines	Unlimited	Number Not Stated	Other
28		6			
29		20			
30			√		
31				√ (> 10)	
32			√		
33			√		
34		20			
35		5			
36			√		(Signalled by + after line #)
37		10			
38			√		
39		20			
40		20			
41		20			
42		20			
43		20			
44		6			
45		10			
46		10			
47		10			
48	√				
49		5			
50		10			
51		5			
52		10			
53		10			
54		10			
55		20			
56		20			
57			√		
58			√		
59		5			
60		20			

TABLE 1 (*continued*)

	Not Permitted	Maximum Total Lines	Unlimited	Number Not Stated	Other
61		20			
62	√				
63		20			
64		20			
65			√		But maximum 330 characters
66			√		
67			√		
68			√		
69			√		
70		20			
71				√	
72				√	
73			√		
74			√		
75		20			
76		20			
77				√	
78		10			But maximum 660 characters
79		20			

program may be entered by passing it electronically from a permanent storage area (a disk, drum, or tape) into the computer's core storage.

Compilation

When the compiler program has been entered into core storage, the FORTRAN program itself may be entered. The computer, acting on the instructions contained in the compiler program, translates each FORTRAN statement to the computer's machine language. In systems with sufficient storage this machine language translation is stored, as it is produced, either in primary or in secondary storage. In smaller systems the machine language translation is delivered as a new deck of punched cards (or reel of tape).

Some terminology and an important distinction are now in order. The program written in FORTRAN language is called the *source* program. The machine language translation produced from it is called the *object* program. The process of translation is called *compilation*. During compilation translated instructions are either stored or delivered as output, but no attempt to *execute* the instructions is being made at this time! In our sample program, the second statement calls for a multiplication. During compilation, this statement generates a digital machine language code signifying multiplication, but no multiplication takes place. Our sample worker's total pay cannot be found anywhere in storage or object program, at the end of this stage. Similarly, the output statement ("WRITE") does not activate any output device during compilation.

Error Messages

One very helpful form of output (in addition to delivery of the translation) does take place during compilation. When any source program statement that contains erroneous FORTRAN language is encountered, the compiler program directs the output of an error message that generally contains (*a*) identification of the statement in the source program that contains the error (and therefore cannot be translated) and (*b*) an error code that may be looked up in a prepared table supplied by the compiler author. For example, if the second statement of our program were mispunched,

$$PAY = 38.0 = 3.17$$

an error message indicating violation of a language rule would be produced. When any language error is found, suitable corrections must be made (by changing one or more cards of the source program), and the entire compilation process must be repeated. Physical delivery of an object program usually stops when any such error is encountered; but the compilation process proceeds to the end of the source program, so that the programmer gets a full list of errors.[1] Since any part of the object program already produced is useless, some compilers provide for a preliminary process called *precompiling*, in which the source program is examined for language errors, and error messages are delivered, with no attempt at physical production of an object program.

---

[1] An unfortunate exception is that some compilers fail to detect a *second* error in a statement already found to contain one mistake.

Execution

When an error-free compilation has been achieved, the programmer's translated instructions are ready for *execution*. If the system provides for storage of the object program during compilation, this execution may be initiated by pushing a console button or by inserting a single instruction statement. If the system is one in which an object deck (punched cards containing the object program) has been produced, this deck must be loaded (i.e., its machine language instructions read into primary storage) before execution can commence.

During execution, the programmer's instructions are followed from top to bottom (unless the programmer has provided "branch" instructions, which we shall introduce shortly). At this stage, another set of error messages may be forthcoming. Though the source program has been proved free of language errors during compilation, certain mistakes in *logic*, or unexpected *data* values,

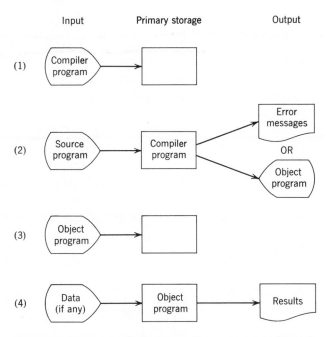

FIG. 10 The compilation-execution sequence. Step 2: compilation; step 4: execution. If sufficient secondary storage is available, steps 1 and 3 do not require card-handling; only source program, data, and some system control cards are loaded for each program.

can render execution of particular instructions impossible. Some examples are attempts to divide by zero or to find the square root of a negative number. The compilation-execution sequence is illustrated in Fig. 10.

In our sample program,

```
C        TOTAL PAY
         PAY = 38.0 * 3.17
         WRITE (3,100) PAY
100      FORMAT (5F15.5)
         END
```

only two statements, the second and third, are *executable* statements. The total effect of the program will be the output of a single number, 120.46000. We shall now examine the program statement by statement.

Comment Statements

The compiler program is prepared to ignore any statement that begins (column 1 of the punched card) with the letter C, which stands for Comment. Thus a Comment statement is not executable, and in fact is not used during compilation either, since no attempt at translation is made. Consequently, you can write (punch) anything you please in such a statement, without regard to FORTRAN language rules.

The Comment statement is intended for the convenience of the programmer. The inclusion of such a statement at the head of a source program ensures that all such card decks (and all listings made from them) will be readily identifiable. Since any number of Comment statements may appear anywhere in the source program, two other uses are also recommended practice. First, early Comment statements may provide explanatory information—author's name, required form of input data, necessary switch settings, and so on. Second, in lengthy programs Comment statements should appear frequently as section headings, so that the programmer (or reader) may locate particular sections easily, and follow the general outline of the program's logic.

Variables and Constants

The second statement in the TOTAL PAY program is an *arithmetic statement*. Arithmetic statements are executable—and in fact are the statements that actually call on the computer to perform its fundamental job: computation.

An arithmetic statement is composed of variables, constants, and operator symbols.[2]

A *variable* is any value in the program designated by the programmer with an alphabetic name. A *constant* is any value introduced within the source program as an actual number. Thus the statement we are examining contains one variable (PAY) and two constants. The rules for assigning names to variables are as follows:

1. The variable name must *begin* with an alphabetic character. Temporarily, however, we rule out six letters of the alphabet—I, J, K, L, M, and N—as permissible *first* characters. Variable names beginning with these "IN-letters" are used in FORTRAN to represent *integer* quantities. When integer variable names (i.e., names starting with I, J, K, L, M, or N) are used by the programmer, the compiler reserves locations that (*a*) cannot hold fractional (postdecimal) portions of values and (*b*) can hold only rather small numbers. For both reasons, *computation* with such variables is risky. They are quite useful, however, for counting purposes and for some specialized computation techniques, which will be discussed in Chapter 5.

2. The other characters that make up the name may be either alphabetic or numerical, but special characters are not usable. Some examples:

Valid Names	Invalid Names	
PAYROL	B1.23	(contains special character)
COST	3XYZ	(begins with numeric character)
SUM3	A+B	(contains special character)
X	ITEM	(temporarily; begins with "IN-letter")
X45		
BC		

3. Maximum length of the variable name varies in different FORTRAN compilers (see Table 2); the most common limitation is six characters (note the odd spelling of the first sample name above).

Given the freedom to choose among billions of possible names, you should immediately adopt the practice of inventing names that are meaningful to you within the context of the program. This facilitates keeping track of the variables as you write the program and also makes later reading much easier (especially for the purpose of locating errors). Thus

$$COST = QUANT * PRICE$$

---

[2] Function names may also appear. They are discussed in Chapter 3.

TABLE 2

Variable Names

	Maximum Number of Characters	Extra Characters May Appear (Are Ignored)	Number Not Stated
1[a]	5		
2	6		
3	6		
4	6		
5	6		
6	6		
7	6		
8	6		
9	8		
10	6		
11	8		
12	8		
13	8		
14	7		
15	7		
16	6		
17	6		
18	5		
19	4		
20	4	√	
21	6		
22	6	√	
23			√
24			√
25	6	√	
26	6		
27	6		
28	6		
29	6		
30	6		

[a] Compiler number.

TABLE 2 (*continued*)

	Maximum Number of Characters	Extra Characters May Appear (Are Ignored)	Number Not Stated
31	12		
32	6		
33	6		
34	6		
35	6		
36	30		
37	6		
38	6		
39	6		
40	6		
41	6		
42	6		
43	6		
44	5		
45	6		
46	6		
47	6		
48	5		
49	5		
50	6		
51	6		
52	6		
53	6		
54	6		
55	6		
56	32		
57	6		
58	6		
59	8	✓	
60	8	✓	
61	6		
62	7	✓	
63	6		

TABLE 2 (*continued*)

	Maximum Number of Characters	Extra Characters May Appear (Are Ignored)	Number Not Stated
64	6		
65	6		
66	6		
67	6		
68	8	√	
69	8	√	
70	6		
71	6		
72	6		
73	6		
74	6		
75	6		
76	6		
77	6		
78	6		
79	6		

is a better statement than an alternative,

$$C = Q * P$$

In writing *constants*, for the moment we shall rule that a decimal point must be written (punched), even for values without fractional content, for constants used in arithmetic statements. The reason is closely connected with our temporary avoidance of the integer *variable*—for under certain circumstances integer constants (written without decimal points) cannot be used successfully in computation.

Storage Locations

Each variable name used by the programmer actually represents a separate storage location. During compilation, each new name mentioned initiates the reservation of an empty location, which will be filled with digital values during execution. This location, which in machine language has a numerical "address," will be catalogued by the compiler program, so that the proper numerical address will be referenced whenever this variable name is mentioned. Thus during compilation of the sample program the first mention of PAY causes a location to be reserved for any numerical values of PAY that may develop during execution. Subsequent mentions (e.g., in the WRITE statement) do not have this effect, but generate machine language instructions containing the correct address for PAY, determined earlier.

It is very important to note that the PAY location is not actually *filled* during compilation. Instructions for filling it are translated to machine language as part of the object program, but have not yet been executed, when compilation is completed.

Basic Arithmetic

The arithmetic statement in the sample program contains, in addition to the variable and two constants, a *replacement symbol* (=) and an *arithmetic operator* (∗).

The sign '=' must appear once, and only once, in every arithmetic statement. Furthermore, to its left must appear *only a single variable name*, nothing more and nothing less. The meaning of the equality symbol in FORTRAN may be paraphrased as follows: "Perform all operations that follow '=' (including looking up mentioned variables in storage and performing arithmetic operations as called for), and place the result in the storage location named on the left of '=.'" The term *replacement* signifies that values previously in that location are now replaced with the new result. Four important points should be noted:

1. If a program's first mention of a variable name should occur on the *right* side of an arithmetic statement, the programmer is committing a grievous error (listed in most error codes as "undefined variable"). He is calling for look-up of a location that cannot yet contain a numerical value! A variable must be *defined* (provided with a numerical value) before it is referred to at the right of an equality symbol. A basic method of defining the variable is by mentioning it on the *left* side of an arithmetic statement.[3]

$$X = 2.4$$

is valid. Further on in the same program,

$$Y = X + 3.$$

is valid, since X has already been defined.

---

[3] Another method is the introduction of the variable in an input list. This will be discussed in Chapter 4.

2. The variable to the left of the equality symbol thus represents a storage location about to be filled or about to have its current value replaced (as soon as the right-side instructions have been followed). But variables mentioned to the *right* of the replacement symbol are looked up and their current values used, without alteration of the location's contents. Thus the value of X in storage remains 2.4 after execution of the last sample statement. If a succeeding statement said

$$X = Y$$

then *both* locations would contain 5.4.

3. To the right of the equality symbol appears an *arithmetic expression*. An arithmetic expression is made up of one or more constants and/or variables, separated by arithmetic operators, function titles, and parentheses. (Functions and parentheses are discussed in Chapter 3.)

4. Everything we have said renders legal an important type of FORTRAN statement that would be nonsense in ordinary algebra. For example,

$$X = X + 1.$$

is perfectly valid, producing *incrementation* of the value stored as X.

Arithmetic Operators

The four operations of simple arithmetic are called for as follows:

+	add
−	subtract
/	divide
*	multiply

Any number of operators[4] may appear in an arithmetic expression. Thus

$$W = G/7. + 2. * A$$

is valid. The order of execution within such a statement will be discussed in Chapter 3. We may observe here, however, that the order follows closely the usual rules of algebra; therefore the statement above is interpreted as

$$w = \frac{g}{7} + 2a$$

Arithmetic operators may not appear in succession in expressions. Thus

$$X = A * -B$$

---

[4] Another arithmetic operator, **, will be discussed in Chapter 3.

will be rejected during compilation. This prohibition usually includes the equality sign, so that

$$V = -X$$

is also illegal. Both statements may be rescued by the use of parentheses:

$$X = A * (-B)$$
$$V = (-X)$$

Output Statements

The third statement in the sample program is an output statement, written in the form appropriate for most current FORTRAN compilers. Output statements are executable, and it should be obvious that one or more of them appears in every program—answers are of no use locked away in storage.

The first number in the parentheses designates the *unit of output equipment* that is to be used; the second is a *statement number*, which refers to the FORMAT statement. The purpose of the FORMAT statement is specification by the programmer of the precise form of the desired output.

The parentheses are followed by the output *list*, which in this instance contains only one variable. Note that an output list can contain *only* variable names, which must be separated by commas.

$$\text{WRITE (3,100) QUANT, PRICE, COST}$$

is valid, but

$$\text{WRITE (3,100) 1952, X, A+B}$$

is not, for the first list item is a constant and the third contains an arithmetic operator.

Each variable mentioned in the output list is looked up, and its current value reproduced by the specified output equipment. The order of reproduction follows the order of listing.

Some other forms of the output statement appear frequently in FORTRAN compilers. For example,

$$\text{WRITE (3) PAY}$$

omits the FORMAT statement number, indicating that the value(s) transmitted are to be reproduced on the output medium in the same form in which they are internally stored (e.g., in binary code).

TABLE 3

Output Statements   (u = equipment unit number;   f = FORMAT statement number)

	WRITE (u,f)	WRITE (u)	PUNCH f	PRINT f	TYPE f	WRITE OUTPUT TAPE u,f	WRITE TAPE u (PAPER TAPE)	PUNCH TAPE f (PAPER TAPE)	PUNCH	PRINT	OTHER
1[a]	✓	✓	.								
2	✓	✓									
3	✓	✓									
4	✓	✓	✓	✓							
5	✓	✓	✓	✓							
6	✓	✓	✓	✓							
7			✓								OUTPUT
8			✓	✓	WRITE TYPE f	✓	✓				PUNCH FLEX f
9		✓	✓	✓		✓	✓				
10	✓	✓	✓	✓		✓	✓				
11	✓	✓	✓	✓		✓	✓				
12	✓	✓	✓	✓		✓	✓				
13	✓	✓	✓	✓		✓	✓				
14	✓	✓	✓	✓			✓				
15	✓	✓	✓	✓			✓				
16			✓	✓		✓	✓				
17		✓	✓	✓		✓	✓				
18	✓	✓	✓	✓						✓	
19		✓									PRINT f, BUFF
20	✓				✓						WRITE, u, b, f
21		✓									[b = TAPE BLOCK #]
22	✓	✓	✓	✓	✓						
23	✓	✓	✓		✓			✓			
24	✓	✓	✓	✓	✓						

[a] Compiler number.

WRITE u

TYPE
WOT u, f

PUNCH (u) f
PRINT (u) f
WRITE
WRITE f (TO FILE)

25
26
27

28
29
30

31
32
33

34

35

36

37
38
39

40
41
42

43
44
45

46
47
48

49
50
51

52
53
54

TABLE 3 (*continued*)

	WRITE (u,f)	WRITE (u)	PUNCH f	PRINT f	TYPE f	WRITE OUTPUT TAPE u,f	WRITE TAPE u	PUNCH TAPE f (PAPER TAPE)	PUNCH	PRINT	OTHER
55	✓	✓	✓	✓							
56	✓	✓								✓	
57	✓		✓	✓					✓	✓	
58	✓		✓	✓							
59	✓	✓	✓	✓	✓	✓	✓	✓			
60	✓	✓	✓	✓							
61	✓	✓	✓	✓							
62		✓	✓	✓					✓	✓	
63		✓	✓	✓							
64	✓	✓	✓	✓		✓	✓				
65	✓	✓	✓	✓							
66	✓	✓	✓	✓					✓	✓	
67	✓	✓	✓	✓	✓						OUTPUT (u)[b]
68	✓	✓	✓	✓	✓						OUTPUT (u)[b]
69	✓	✓									
70	✓	✓	✓	✓							
71	✓	✓									
72	✓	✓									
73	✓	✓	✓	✓		✓	✓		✓		
74	✓	✓	✓	✓		✓					
75	✓	✓	✓	✓					✓	✓	WRITE OUTPUT TAPE u
76	✓	✓	✓	✓		✓	✓				
77	✓	✓	✓	✓		✓	✓				
78	✓	✓	✓	✓		✓	✓				
79	✓	✓									

[b] List may include arithmetic expressions.

In older FORTRAN versions ("FORTRAN II") the word WRITE is frequently replaced by PRINT (referring to a console typewriter or on-line printer), PUNCH (referring to card output), or TYPE (console typewriter), accompanied by a FORMAT statement number, but no equipment unit number:

> PRINT 100, PAY
>
> PUNCH 100, PAY
>
> TYPE 100, PAY

The PRINT and PUNCH forms also appear in some later compilers ("FORTRAN IV"), to refer to an on-line printer and punched cards, respectively.

Output statements are also used that refer specifically to *tape* output:

> WRITE OUTPUT TAPE 7,100, PAY
>
> or   WRITE TAPE 7, PAY

The first example refers to tape unit number 7 and provides a FORMAT reference. The second is "unformatted," indicating transmission in internal storage form.

Table 3 shows the permissible output statement forms for various FORTRAN compilers. Equipment reference numbers vary with system configurations[5] and are frequently assigned by the individual installation; consult your computer center staff.

FORMAT Statements

The FORMAT statement is nonexecutable. It can actually be placed almost anywhere in the source program (except after END), since it is really bypassed during execution and referred to only when mentioned in an input or output statement.

The FORMAT statement must be numbered. (We discuss statement numbers later in this chapter.) The word FORMAT is followed by parentheses, which contain precise instructions for form of output, including

> vertical position
> horizontal position
> type of notation (e.g., decimal, exponential, integer)
> number of decimal places
> alphabetic titles

---

[5] "Configuration" is trade jargon translating roughly as "equipment collection."

Since the design of output can be complicated, we are going to postpone the subject for a considerable period while we work on the basic techniques of computation. Therefore, in your first programs simply reproduce the FORMAT statement in the TOTAL PAY program

100   FORMAT (5F15.5)

and use the number 100 in all output statements (and in input statements, when we begin using them). Thus your early programs will produce output in a standard format, which contains up to five values per line, unlabeled, each with five decimal places. Each output value occupies a space 15 characters in width.

The END Statement

The word END *must* appear at the end of every source program. It is not an executable statement, but is necessary during compilation, to tell the compiler that all program statements have now been read. When END is encountered, the compiler program usually produces a message indicating that compilation has been completed.

Statement Numbers

When a statement is to be numbered by the programmer, the number must appear within the first five columns of the card (coding paper). A statement number *cannot* have a decimal point. Most FORTRAN compilers permit numbers between 1 and 99999. Some have a lower limit, as noted in Table 4.

TABLE 4

Statement Numbers—Maximum Value

	9999	32767	99999	Other
1[a]	√			
2			√	
3			√	
4			√	
5			√	
6			√	
7				2047
8			√	
9			√	

[a] Compiler number.

TABLE 4 (*continued*)

	9999	32767	99999	Other
10			√	
11		√		
12		√		
13			√	
14			√	
15			√	
16			√	
17			√	
18	√			
19	√			
20				2047
21			√	
22			√	
23			√	
24		√		
25			√	
26			√	
27			√	
28			√	
29			√	
30			√	
31		√		
32			√	
33		√		
34			√	
35			√	
36			√	or alphabetic label followed by colon
37			√	
38			√	
39			√	
40			√	
41				65535
42			√	
43			√	
44			√	
45			√	

TABLE 4 (*continued*)

	9999	32767	99999	Other
46			√	
47			√	
48	√			
49			√	
50			√	
51			√	
52			√	
53			√	
54			√	
55		√		
56			√	
57			√	
58			√	
59			√	
60			√	
61		√		
62			√	
63			√	
64			√	
65			√	
66			√	
67			√	
68			√	
69			√	
70			√	
71		√		
72			√	
73			√	
74			√	
75			√	
76		√		
77		√		
78		√		
79				"5 digits"

Most statements do not *require* numbering. The FORMAT statement is an exception, since it must always be referenced by input and output statements. A statement number is generally used *only* when the statement being written is to be referred to by another statement. When statement numbers are used, they need not be in sequence and need not represent actual card position in any way. The only consistency required is that between a statement's number and the number mentioned in the statement designed to refer to it.

The freedom to choose statement numbers arbitrarily becomes valuable in complex programs, for it permits insertion of numbers as afterthoughts, without alteration of numbers already used. Thus in the segment

```
            _____
23          _____
            _____
24          _____
240         _____
25          _____
```

the insertion of number 240 is perfectly valid. However, many programmers follow the practice of numbering at intervals of ten, to preserve statement number sequence after insertions are made. They would have written

```
230         _____
            _____
240         _____
241         _____
250         _____
```

A Branch Statement

You surely have the feeling that our first program underutilizes the computer's capabilities. The execution is over in a blinding flash, but the overall time including writing, keypunching, and compiling is hardly impressive in light of the fact that an electric calculator or pencil and paper would be faster for the problem as stated. Furthermore, the program is useless for problems other than the very particular one for which it was written.

The computer becomes really useful—its "comparative advantage" is highest, the economist would say—when a *repetitive* process is required. For this reason, almost every useful computer program contains at least one *branch statement.* The computer's performance will outdistance the electric calculator by a great margin if we turn the TOTAL PAY question into a table-producing program. Let us write a program that will produce as output the total pay owed at the $3.17 wage rate, for each possible number of whole hours worked (hours also to be shown in output).

```
C       PAY TABLE FOR $3.17 WAGE RATE
100     FORMAT (5F15.5)
        HOURS = 1.0
38    ⌈PAY = HOURS * 3.17
      │WRITE (3,100) HOURS, PAY
      │HOURS = HOURS + 1.0
      ⌊GO TO 38
        END
```

The statement

$$GO\ TO\ \#$$

is an *unconditional branch* statement. Any branch instruction causes the computer to depart from its top-to-bottom execution of statements, branching back *or* forward to the statement whose number is mentioned. This one provides no alternative routes—hence the description as unconditional.

The program contains a *loop*, a technique that lies at the heart of all programming. The bracket drawn on the left to show the *range* of the loop is common practice for the programmer's convenience in writing and reading the program. It has no FORTRAN meaning, since it cannot be keypunched. (The next sample program uses *indentation* of repeated statements as an interesting alternative, to improve readability.)

The number following GO TO must be a statement number; it must be matched by a number appearing somewhere in the program in the first five columns, attached to an *executable* statement.

The loop in the PAY TABLE program is *endless*, since the repetition of the two arithmetic, one output, and one branch statement has not been limited in any way by the programmer. This program can be stopped by manual control at the computer console (always equipped with a simple STOP button). The programmer can control the number of repetitions in a loop only by using some form of *conditional* branch statement, a subject introduced in Chapter 4.

One of the important operations that may be accomplished by a loop is *summation.* For example, the following program prints the successive sums of integers 1 through n (the ultimate value of n depending on when the STOP button is pushed):

```
C       SUMS OF INTEGERS
100     FORMAT (5F15.5)
        SUM = 0.
        XNUM = 1.
333         SUM = SUM + XNUM
            WRITE (3,100) XNUM, SUM
            XNUM = XNUM + 1.0
            GO TO 333
        END
```

Notice the necessity for defining the SUM (as zero) *before* its appearance on the right side of an arithmetic statement. This is frequently referred to as *initialization*; it avoids the error "undefined variable." The first execution of the summation statement cannot be properly performed without prior initialization. Note also the form of the summation and incrementation statements, both of which logically require the mention of a variable name on *both* sides of the replacement symbol (=).

For the sample program, you should be able to verify that the two storage locations used are filled during execution as follows:

	SUM	XNUM
preloop (1)	0.	empty
preloop (2)	0.	1.
3)	1.	1.
4)	1.	2.
5)	3.	2.
6)	3.	3.
7)	6.	3.
8)	6.	4.
9)	10.	4.

etc.

Before you attempt the first set of exercises, heed some important injunctions:

1. Since you are learning a *language*, you cannot complete the learning process by reading only. Conversation practice is essential, and this conversation must take place between you and the computer. Many alternative problems, drawn from a variety of subject areas, are presented for exercise following each

chapter, so that you may be selective according to your interests—but *do* write a few programs from every exercise set! (Sufficient technical information—such as formulas—is provided with each exercise to permit completion without prior knowledge of the discipline represented.)

2. You must do more than write the programs. Have them keypunched and run them on the computer. The *debugging* process, in which you respond to the computer's error messages denoting language errors, or to wrong answers resulting from logical errors (by making suitable corrections and trying again), utilizes the computer as a sort of teaching machine. Furthermore, for complex problems, a successful run on the computer is the *only* acceptable evidence that a program is correctly written. Experienced programmers heed the first axiom of computer programming, which derives from Murphy's law:[6] "There is at least one error in every program."

3. To facilitate the testing and debugging process, Appendix A contains a uniform trial data set and correct output values for all exercise programs. Since there are usually dozens, occasionally millions, of alternative methods of writing a computer program to solve a given problem, Appendix A represents the only sort of "answer" key you should need. Any program that produces correct output is a correct program. The absence of error messages does not guarantee freedom from logic errors—so check carefully.

4. *A technical note on endless loops:* The first two exercise sets (Chapters 2 and 3) suggest programs that can be written in the manner of our last two examples (PAY TABLE, SUMS OF INTEGERS). The *endless* loop, however, is a technique that we shall soon abandon completely, since (*a*) *infinite* repetition is not required, in real problems, and (*b*) the endless loop can create a control problem at the computer console during execution.

If you are present during running of your programs, you may terminate the execution by using console buttons. (Incidentally, your presence is highly desirable for other reasons: debugging may require several compilation and execution attempts for each program; the process becomes inefficient when conducted *in absentia*, by examination of delivered output.) If, however, you will not be present, the computer operator should be warned when your programs contain endless loops, so that he may take appropriate action. At installations that stack programs for "batch processing" your endless loop may require use of a time-limit method of terminating execution and/or the use of special control cards ahead of the following program. The question should be discussed with computer personnel.

---

[6] Murphy's law states: "If anything can go wrong, it will."

If the endless loop creates insurmountable problems, here is a solution that will not be fully explained until Chapter 5. To limit output from each such program to *twenty* lines, keypunch this card:

DO 99 K = 1, 20

Use the card as follows:

1. Place the DO statement *ahead of* the *first* executable statement of your loop.

2. Label as statement 99 the *last* executable statement of your loop.

3. Omit the GO TO statement.

For example, for our last program,

```
333   ⎡ SUM = SUM + XNUM              ⎡ DO 99 K = 1,20
      ⎮ WRITE (3,100) XNUM, SUM       ⎮ SUM = SUM + XNUM
      ⎮ XNUM = XNUM + 1.0             ⎮ WRITE (3,100) XNUM, SUM
      ⎣ GO TO 333                  99 ⎣ XNUM = XNUM + 1.0
```

(The statement number 333 is no longer needed. For most compilers, however, the result of leaving it in would be an error message during compilation ("unreferenced statement number 333"), which would *not* prevent full production of the object program.)

For Review	Examples
FORTRAN coding form	
statement continuation	
source program	
object program	
compilation	
execution	
error messages	
precompiling	
executable statement	
Comment statement	C THIS IS A COMMENT
variable	A, BAKER
constant	3.2, 4.
IN-letters	I, J, K, L, M, N
arithmetic statement	A = B + C
replacement symbol	=
undefined variable	
arithmetic operator	+ − * /
arithmetic expression	B + C/2.

For Review   **Examples**

incrementation $X = X + 1.0$

output statement   WRITE (3,100) A, B, C

output list   A, B, C

FORMAT statement   100   FORMAT (5F15.5)

END statement   END

branch statement

unconditional branch statement   GO TO 10

loop

endless loop

initialization   SUM = 0.

summation   SUM = SUM + X

debugging

EXERCISES

1. Write a program that will produce a multiplication table for the number **13**.

2. If the "consumption function" of economic theory says

    consumer expenditure = **78.3** + **0.83** (income)

    write a program that will produce a table of consumer expenditures for incomes of 100, 110, 120, 130, etc.

3. An object dropped from a height travels the distance

    $$d = \tfrac{1}{2}at^2$$

    where a = **32.16** (ft/sec^2; the gravitational constant) and t = time in seconds. Write a program that will generate a table of distances for times of 1 second, 3 seconds, 5 seconds, 7 seconds, etc.

4. The speed of a chemical reaction *doubles* for every 10 degree (Centigrade) rise in temperature. At 0°C the reaction time is 3414 seconds. Write a program that will generate a table showing the reaction time for 10°, 20°, 30°, 40°, etc. Output should include temperatures and times.

5. Given the length (l) of a simply supported beam, and a uniform load (w), *shear* and *moment* are dependent on the load's distance (x) from the beginning of the span:

    $$shear = \frac{wl}{2} - wx$$

    $$moment = \frac{wlx}{2} - \frac{wx^2}{2}$$

Write a program that, for a 50-foot beam and uniform load 1000 pounds per foot, will compute *shear* and *moment* for distances 0 feet, 5 feet, 10 feet, 15 feet, 20 feet, etc.

6. The geometric constant π (3.1415927) can be found by evaluating the series:

$$4 - {}^4/_3 + {}^4/_5 - {}^4/_7 + {}^4/_9 \cdots$$

Write an "endless loop" program to evaluate the series. (*Hint:* each time through the loop, compute and output *two* additional terms.)

7. If W_1 and W_2 represent two weights to be placed on a meter stick, and D_1 and D_2 their respective distances from the pivot point, a basic principle in the mechanics of solids says that balance requires

$$W_1D_1 + W_2D_2 = 0$$

A 17-ounce weight is to be placed opposite a 13-ounce weight. Write a program that will compute the appropriate distance for the 17-ounce weight, for various placements of the 13-ounce weight: -1 cm, -2 cm, -3 cm, -4 cm, etc.

8. An item is to be sold for either $6.49 or $7.98. Write a program that will produce a table showing on each line total revenue at each price, from the sale of 12 units, 24 units, 36 units, etc.

9. An airliner travels at the speed of 307.45 miles per hour. Write a program that will produce a table of distances covered in 5 minutes, 10 minutes, 15 minutes, 20 minutes, etc.

10. Seventy-nine consumers are to be asked a question. Write a program that will prepare a presurvey table showing all possible *percentages* who may say "Yes."

11. Write a program that will produce a table of *factorial* numbers (n! = 1 × 2 × 3 × 4 ⋯ × n) beginning with 1!, 2!, 3!, 4!, etc.

3 • EXPANSION OF COMPUTATION TECHNIQUES

The four basic operations of arithmetic are each translated by most compilers to a single machine language code. Thus addition, multiplication, subtraction, and division are fundamental activities for which most modern computers are prepared by their *hardware*. The FORTRAN compiler (a valuable piece of *software*) provides certain computation routines that enable the programmer to call for some complex arithmetic operations, without providing detailed instructions. That is, the compiler will respond to a single FORTRAN word or symbol by generating a *sequence* of machine language statements.

Exponentiation

One of the computational symbols, ∗∗, is officially classified as an *arithmetic operator*, because it may be used in the same manner, as +, −, /, and ∗. That is, the double asterisk appears in arithmetic expressions between any two values (which may be variables, constants, or arithmetic expressions combining variables and constants). It specifies exponentiation; for example, X^{12} is computed by writing

$$X**12.0$$

Some examples of exponentiation:

	Algebraic	FORTRAN
(1)	a^3	A∗∗3
(2)	$g + h^2$	G + H∗∗2
(3)	$(r + s)^5$	(R + S)∗∗5
(4)	4^d	4.∗∗D
(5)	v^x	V∗∗X
(6)	X^{378}	X∗∗378.
(7)	$b^{5.6}$	B∗∗5.6
(8)	$w^{1/3}$	W∗∗(1./3.)

Examples 3 and 8 make use of parentheses, in the former to *group* terms for the *argument* and in the latter to do the same for the *exponent*. As in algebra, parentheses in FORTRAN are used to indicate precedence of enclosed operations. Execution order within arithmetic expressions is discussed later in this chapter. Here we may note, however, that the removal of parentheses in these two instances would produce:

$$(3) \qquad r + s^5$$

$$(8) \qquad \frac{w^1}{3}$$

In the first three examples, the decimal point has been omitted from the exponent. This is an exception to a rule adopted in Chapter 2 for constants in arithmetic statements. It is not only permissible to omit decimal points in *exponents*, but desirable in many instances. The reason is that most FORTRAN compilers will interpret the nondecimal exponent as calling for straight multiplication. For example,

G**3

is compiled and executed as

G * G * G

But if a decimal point appears in the exponent, the compiler produces a method employing logarithms. Therefore

G**3.

is compiled and executed as

antilog(3log g)

or as the programmer might have written it in FORTRAN (after reading the next section),

EXP(3.*ALOG(G))

Since the approximation of the logarithm produces rounding error, small exponents are frequently written without decimals; but large exponents written without decimal points are costly in terms of execution time. For instance, X^{1774} should be written

X**1774.

as in the example 6 above.[1] Note, however, that *negative* arguments cannot have decimal exponents, since logarithms cannot be obtained for negative numbers. Thus

$$(-3.)**55.$$

is not valid, but

$$(-3.)**55$$

may be used.

The decimal point should *not* be excluded from the *argument* (the number to be raised to a power), as shown in example 4. Instances in which the decimal point is mandatory for the *exponent* are shown in examples 7 and 8. In example 7 this is true simply because the exponent has decimal content to begin with. In example 8 arithmetic is being called for to evaluate the exponent, hence the usual rule regarding constants in arithmetic expressions must be followed. Observe that what is being computed in this example is the cube root. Some alternatives to the SQRT function (discussed below) are then evidently

$$X**(1./2.)$$
$$\text{or} \quad X**.5$$

FORTRAN-Supplied Functions

In the preceding section we have mentioned several FORTRAN words—EXP, ALOG, SQRT—which call for multistep arithmetic procedures. The FORTRAN compiler provides computation routines for many mathematical functions which are useful in a wide variety of problems. These may appear in arithmetic expressions. The function title is followed by parentheses that contain the *argument*—the value on which the required computation is to be performed.

The argument itself is an arithmetic expression and therefore may be a single variable or constant, or combinations of these separated as usual by arithmetic operators, parentheses, and other function titles. Functions may be used only on the *right* side of arithmetic statements (i.e., within arithmetic

---

[1] Some compilers automatically resort to the logarithmic procedure for exponents larger than a fixed limit, effectively ignoring the decimal point in such cases.

expressions). As usual, the values of variables mentioned (as arguments) are not altered by the process.

The functions supplied by most FORTRAN compilers include:[2]

SQRT( )	square root
ABS( )	absolute value
ALOG( )	logarithm (base e)
EXP( )	antilogarithm (base e)
ALOG10( )	logarithm (base 10)
SIN( )	sine
COS( )	cosine
ATAN( )	arctangent

Square Root

Neither computer nor compiler contains prepared tables of such functions as square roots, logarithms, cosines, and so on. Each of these functions is approximated by a computation routine, which is generated in machine language when the programmer uses the appropriate FORTRAN word (function title). Thus "SQRT" acts as a convenient substitute for a whole series of FORTRAN statements that might be written by the programmer who remembers how to obtain a square root by some method employing addition, subtraction, multiplication, and division. The parentheses following each function word indicate the extent of the argument and must appear even when the argument is a single variable or constant. Some examples:

Algebraic	FORTRAN
$\sqrt{2a}$	SQRT(2.*A)
$\sqrt{b^3}$	SQRT(B**3)
$4\sqrt{w}$	4.*SQRT(W)
$\sqrt{g + h}$	SQRT(G + H)
$\sqrt{g} + h$	SQRT(G) + H
$\sqrt{\log_e g}$	SQRT(ALOG(G))

---

[2] Not a complete list; others will be listed and discussed in Chapters 9 and 10.

Absolute Value

This function obtains the value of the argument, disregarding sign. Thus the result is the same as the argument, if the latter is positive; but for negative arguments, the result is positive.

Algebraic	FORTRAN
$\lvert x \rvert$	ABS(X)
$\lvert a - b \rvert$	ABS(A − B)
$\lvert v \rvert^{10.2}$	(ABS(V)∗∗10.2)

Logarithms

Since the computer multiplies and divides very rapidly, you should certainly not resort to logarithms merely as a computation alternative. For example, it would be foolish to substitute for

$$A = B*C/D$$

by writing

$$A = EXP(ALOG(B) + ALOG(C) - ALOG(D))$$

The latter would be slower in execution, as well as bulkier to write and keypunch and more likely to produce rounding error in answers. Even for instances in which you would be forced to use logarithms in hand computation, shorthand alternatives are preferable in FORTRAN. Thus

$$a^{1/6} \quad (\text{or } \sqrt[6]{a})$$

can be written

$$A**(1./6.)$$
$$\text{or} \quad A**.1667$$

There are, however, many problems for which logarithms are essential; some examples are given in the exercises.

The ALOG function produces *natural* logarithms (base e). Some FORTRAN compilers also provide ALOG10, which obtains *common* logarithms (base 10). In other systems, remember that

$$\log_{10} a = \log_e a / \log_e 10$$

and write the conversion into your program when required.

EXP(X) calls for the antilogarithm (base e), which is of course e^x. A function for *common* antilogarithms is usually not provided. However, from the definition of the logarithm, the programmer who wants antilog$_{10}$ X merely writes 10.**X.

Algebraic	FORTRAN
log$_e$ x	ALOG(X)
3 log$_e$ d	3.*ALOG(D)
log$_e$ (a + b)	ALOG(A + B)
log$_{10}$ w	ALOG10(W) or ALOG(W)/ALOG(10.)
antilog$_e$ v	EXP(V)
antilog$_{10}$ h	10.**H
e^x	EXP(X)

Trigonometric Functions

The arguments for SIN and COS must be stated in *radians*, and the result of ATAN is returned in radians. The various functions are obtained by approximation routines.

Algebraic	FORTRAN
cos A	COS(A)
r sin G	R * SIN(G)
(cos v)(sin t)	COS(V) * SIN(T)
atan p	ATAN(P)

TABLE 5

FORTRAN-Supplied Functions

	SQRT	ABS	ALOG	EXP	ALOG10	SIN	COS	ATAN
1[a]	✓	✓	✓	✓		✓	✓	✓
2	✓	✓	✓	✓		✓	✓	✓
3	✓	✓	✓	✓	✓	✓	✓	✓
4	✓	✓	✓	✓	✓	✓	✓	✓
5	✓	✓	✓	✓	✓	✓	✓	✓
6	✓	✓	✓	✓	✓	✓	✓	✓
7	SQRTF	ABSF	LOGF	EXPF		SINF	COSF	ATANF
8	SQRTF	ABSF	LOGF	EXPF		SINF	COSF	ATANF
9	SQRTF	ABSF	LOGF	EXPF		SINF	COSF	ATANF

[a] Compiler number.

TABLE 5 (*continued*)

	SQRT	ABS	ALOG	EXP	ALOG10	SIN	COS	ATAN
10	√	√	√	√		√	√	√
11	√	√	√	√		√	√	√
12	√	√	√	√		√	√	√
13	√	√	√	√	√	√	√	√
14	√	√	√	√	√	√	√	√
15	√	√	√	√	√	√	√	√
16	SQRTF	ABSF	LOGF	EXPF	LOG10	SINF	COSF	ATANF
17	√	√	LOG	√		√	√	√
18	√	√	√	√		√	√	√
19				[None]				
20	SQTF		LOGF	EXPF		SINF	COSF	ATNF
21	√	√	√	√	√	√	√	√
22	√	√	√	√	√	√	√	√
23	√	√	√	√	√	√	√	√
24	√	√	√	√	√	√	√	√
25	√	√	√	√	√	√	√	√
26	√	√	√	√		√	√	√
27	SQRTF	ABSF	LOGF	EXPF		SINF	COSF	ATANF
28	√	√	√	√	√	√	√	√
29	√	√	√	√	√	√	√	√
30	√	√	√	√		√	√	√
31	SQRTF	ABSF	LOGF	EXPF		SINF	COSF	ATANF
32	SQRTF	ABSF	LOGF	EXPF		SINF	COSF	ATANF
33	√	√	√	√[b]	√	√	√	√
34	√	√	√	√	√	√	√	√
35	SQRTF	ABSF	LOGF	EXPF		SINF	COSF	ATANF
36	√	√	√	√		√	√	√[c]
37	√	√	√	√	√	√	√	√
38	√	√	√	√	√	√	√	√
39	√	√	√	√	√	√	√	√
40	√	√	√	√	√	√	√	√
41	√	√	√	√	√	√	√	√
42	√	√	√	√	√	√	√	√

[b] Also EXP10.

[c] Also accepts FORTRAN II function titles.

TABLE 5 (*continued*)

	SQRT	ABS	ALOG	EXP	ALOG10	SIN	COS	ATAN
43	√	√	√	√	√	√	√	√
44	√	√	√	√		√	√	√
45	SQRTF	ABSF	LOGF	EXPF		SINF	COSF	ATANF
46	SQRTF	ABSF	LOGF	EXPF		SINF	COSF	ATANF
47	√	√	√	√	√	√	√	√
48	√		√	√		√	√	√
49	√	√	√	√		√	√	√
50	√	√	√	√		√	√	√
51	√	√	√	√	√	√	√	√
52	√	√	√	√	√	√	√	√
53	SQRTF	ABSF	LOGF	EXPF	LOGXF	SINF	COSF	ATANF
54	√	√	√	√	ALOGB	√	√	√
55	√	√	√	√	√	√	√	√
56	√	√	√	√ ^{b}	√	√	√	√
57	SQRTF	ABSF	LOGF	EXPF		SINF	COSF	ATANF
58	SQRTF	ABSF	LOGF	EXPF		SINF	COSF	ATANF
59				[Not stated]				
60	√	√	√	√	√	√	√	√
61	√	√	√	√	√	√	√	√
62	SQRTF	ABSF	LOGF	EXPF		SINF	COSF	ATANF
63	√	√	√	√	√	√	√	√
64	√	√	√	√	√	√	√	√
65	SQRTF	ABSF	LOGF	EXPF		SINF	COSF	ATANF
66	√	√	√	√	√	√	√	√
67	√	√	√	√		√	√	√
68	√	√	√	√	√	√	√	√ ^{c}
69	√	√	√	√	√	√	√	√ ^{c}
70	√	√	√	√	√	√	√	√
71	√	√	√	√	√	√	√	√
72	√	√	√	√	√	√	√	√
73	√	√	√	√	√	√	√	√
74	√	√	√	√	√	√	√	√
75	√	√	√	√ ^{b}	√	√	√	√
76	√	√	√	√	√	√	√	√
77	√	√	√	√	√	√	√	√
78	√	√	√	√ ^{b}	√	√	√	√
79	√	√	√	√	√	√	√	√

Table 5 shows availability of the functions discussed thus far, in various compilers. Note that FORTRAN II function words generally end with the letter F. The list of FORTRAN-supplied functions will be expanded in later chapters (indexed in Tables 19, 21, and 22).

The Importance of Subprograms in Programming

The functions we have just examined are important examples of the *subprogram*, which we may define as *any set of instructions that, once written, may be stored and called into use by name*. Let us pause for a moment to admire the *idea* of subprograms, to make a philosophic observation on the subject, and to foreshadow some later techniques.

The FORTRAN-supplied functions would appear to the computer-center visitor to justify such a statement as "This computer knows how to find a square root." Does the computer "know" any such thing? Of course not. It is the man who wrote the FORTRAN compiler who knows how to obtain a square root. Then what *does* the computer "know"? Not very much; for example, division and multiplication, which most computers accomplish by iterative subtraction and addition, could very well be called *subprograms* written by the computer designer. And in the opposite direction, once you have written a program that performs multiple correlation analysis on any appropriate data set, you might tell the visitor that your computer "knows" how to accomplish multiple correlation. Undue modesty on your part. As we shall see in Chapter 12, complete programs placed in secondary storage can be made to fulfill our *subprogram* definition; they may be called into use by name.

Another important possibility will be fully explored in Chapter 9. Computation routines that you write in FORTRAN may be treated by you subsequently as functions. For example, having written a program that computes the arithmetic mean for any data set, it is possible to assign an alphabetic title to the program and thereafter call forth the entire operation by mentioning that title and providing the arguments (in this instance a series of values) on which the subprogram is to perform.

In this manner, the programmer may build on his previous work, as though the computer "knew" how to do anything that the programmer has had to do at an earlier date.

Before turning to another subject, let us demonstrate the use of some FORTRAN-supplied functions by directing the computer to generate a table of x, x^2, $\sqrt{x}$, $\sqrt{10x}$, and $\log_e x$, for x = 1.0, 1.1, 1.2, 1.3, and so on.

```
C        TABLE OF CERTAIN FUNCTIONS
100      FORMAT (5F15.5)
         X = 1.0
35     ┌ A = X**2
       │ B = SQRT(X)
       │ C = SQRT(10.*X)
       │ D = ALOG(X)
       │ WRITE (3,100) X, A, B, C, D
       │ X = X + 0.1
       └ GO TO 35
         END
```

Compound Arithmetic

Arithmetic expressions can and should be lengthy. A basic advantage of FORTRAN is suggested by its title—the programmer is able to translate any "formula" in its entirety in a single FORTRAN statement. Chopping into segments is not necessary and is in fact poor practice. Thus

$$r_2 = \frac{-b + \sqrt{b^2 - 4ac}}{2a}$$

should be translated to a single FORTRAN statement (assuming, of course, that a, b, and c have been defined earlier in the program). However,

$$R2 = -B + SQRT\ B**2 - 4.*A*C/2.*A$$

is wrong, on several counts.

First, we have already stated that the SQRT function requires parentheses around the entire argument.

$$R2 = -B + SQRT(B**2 - 4.*A*C)/2.*A$$

does not solve the problem completely, however. In its present form, the statement would be executed as

$$-b + \frac{\sqrt{b^2 - 4ac}}{2} \quad (a)$$

Even before discussing FORTRAN execution-order rules, we can solve this problem with a simple corollary of those rules: when dividing, enclose the numerator and/or denominator in parentheses when either contains more than one term. Thus

$$R2 = (-B + SQRT(B**2 - 4.*A*C))/(2.*A)$$

will be properly executed.

The execution-order rules, which are imitative of ordinary practice in algebra, are as follows.

Order of precedence in arithmetic statements:

1. Parentheses (innermost first)
2. Functions (from left to right)
3. ** (from left to right)
4. * and / (equal precedence; from left to right)
5. + and − (equal precedence; from left to right)

In executing

$$V = W + X/Y**B$$

the computer will first evaluate y^b, then evaluate $X/result$, and finally do the addition. This produces

$$v = w + \frac{x}{y^b}$$

If the programmer really wants

$$v = w + (x/y)^b$$

he must write

$$V = W + (X/Y)**B$$

and for

$$v = (w + x/y)^b$$

he writes

$$V = (W + X/Y)**B$$

Finally, for

$$v = \frac{w + x}{y^b}$$

he writes

$$V = (W + X)/Y**B$$

Note that the presence of *extra* parentheses does no damage (so long as they are placed in pairs); therefore when in doubt, use them. For instance, the last statement would execute identically if written

$$V = (W + X)/(Y**B)$$

The trigonometric formula

$$\tan \tfrac{1}{2}\theta = \pm\sqrt{\frac{1 - \cos \theta}{1 + \cos \theta}}$$

would be written,[3] for one result,

$$TAN1 = SQRT((1.-COS(THETA))/(1. + COS(THETA)))$$

Verify that the translation is correct and also that there are no *extra* parentheses in the statement as written.

Note that multiplication and division have *equal* precedence, as do addition and subtraction. The left-to-right rule decides the issue. Thus

$$\frac{a}{bc}$$

cannot be written as

$$A/B*C$$

Remember that in the process of translating from algebra to FORTRAN, you have three other continuing responsibilities:

1. Valid FORTRAN titles must be assigned to all variables. In particular, remember that

$$\overline{X} = \frac{\Sigma X}{n}$$

can get you into trouble if translated

$$XBAR = SUMX/N$$

because the "N" title is reserved by the "IN-letter" rule. Why not XNUM?

2. For much the same reason, remember to insert decimal points for integer constants (optional only for exponents).

3. You must insert operator symbols—avoid a common error, which is to

---

[3] THETA having been defined earlier in the program.

translate 3b into 3.B instead of 3.*B. Implied multiplication is a convention of algebra that is not valid in FORTRAN.

Exponential Notation

Mathematicians, engineers, and others are familiar with the notation

$$3(10)^9$$

to represent

$$3,000,000,000$$

or

$$2(10)^{-5}$$

for

$$.00002$$

The computer will recognize such expressions as valid constants, the form being

$$3.E+9 \quad \text{(or } .3E+10, \text{ etc.)}$$
$$2.E-5 \quad \text{(or } 20.E-6, \text{ etc.)}$$

in which E is shorthand for "exponent of 10." For the uninitiated, note that the exponent may be treated as a simple instruction to move the decimal point a specified number of places to the left ($-$) or right ($+$) of its stated position.

Furthermore, the computer will (at the programmer's instruction) reproduce output in this *exponential* form, so that very large (or very small) numbers may be contained in relatively narrow output fields. Though we do not discuss the method fully until Chapter 6, you may view such output by changing our standard FORMAT statement to read

$$100 \quad \text{FORMAT (5E15.5)}$$

This substitution of "E" for "F" will be suggested in some exercise problems.

Range and Precision of Decimal Values

An important piece of information should now be considered: the computer actually *stores* decimal values by a method utilizing exponential notation. This permits the storage of a large *range* of values in a location of fixed length. In a binary-coded decimal system, for example, the number 15.25 might be stored as

	1	5	2	5	0	0	0	0	0	2
	:	:	:	:	:	:	:	:	:	:
$2^3 = 8\ldots$										
$2^2 = 4\ldots$		x		x						
$2^1 = 2\ldots$			x							x
$2^0 = 1\ldots$	x	x		x						

The system pictured (e.g., IBM 1620) reserves a maximum of eight cells for actual digits of the number and provides two cells (at the extreme right) for the exponent. The decimal point is counted from the left (its position in a *normalized* number), so that the meaning here is

$$.1525(10)^2$$

In such a system the largest number that could be stored would have 99 pre-decimal digits (exponent 99), whereas the smallest (positive) number capable of being stored will contain 99 postdecimal zeroes (exponent -99).

In a straight binary system the same *floating point* method is generally used; both the digital portion (*characteristic*) and the exponent (*mantissa*) are separately held in binary form, and frequently the predecimal and postdecimal portions of the number are separately represented. As an example, the IBM 1130 system would store the number 15.25 in a 32-bit location:

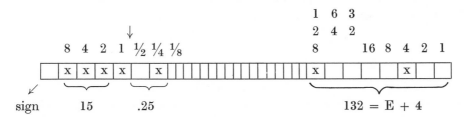

The leftmost bit is reserved for sign of the number ("on" for negative). The exponent appears in the right-hand eight bits and is interpreted by subtracting 128. Thus the "132" in storage signifies "E + 4," which locates the binary point at the position marked by an arrow. To the left of this point,

$$2^0 + 2^1 + 2^2 + 2^3 = 1 + 2 + 4 + 8 = 15.$$

To the right,

$$2^{-2} = \frac{1}{2^2} = \frac{1}{4} = .25$$

Since the range of possible exponents is ± 127, the largest number that could be stored is

$$2^0 + 2^1 + 2^2 + \cdots + 2^{126}$$

which is approximately 10^{38}. The lower limit is of course 10^{-38} (signifying a small *positive* number).

For all systems, then, it is evident that the computer will handle numbers only within some limited range. Values generated by computation that are outside this range (too large or too small to be stored) cause execution error called *overflow* or *underflow* and lead to incorrect output.

A distinction must be made between *range* and *precision* of values. The latter word refers to the *number of digits* that can be accurately stored for any single value, rather than to the maximum numerical quantity that may be represented. For example,

$$1.2345678E + 45$$

represents a very large quantity, but is precise to only eight digits.

While *range* is a function of the permissible size of exponents, *precision* depends on the total storage length (number of "bits") allocated for each value. Most computers operate with a normal precision limit of between seven and twelve digits.[4] In binary-coded decimal systems, nonsignificant (i.e., inaccurate; beyond precision limits) digits in output may show up as zeroes to the right of the postdecimal significant digits. Thus the result of

$$1.E+06/3.0$$

might be printed as

$$333333.33000$$

(using our standard FORMAT statement, which calls for five decimal places in output; the computer used having eight-digit precision). In binary systems the situation is more dangerous for the unwary reader of output, since the result may be nonzero, nonsignificant digits; for example,

$$333333.33589$$

Table 6 shows the maximum range and precision of decimal numbers for various FORTRAN compilers. (The table reflects restraints imposed by the computer for which the compiler is written.)

---

[4] Provisions for extending this precision are discussed in Chapter 10.

TABLE 6

Decimal Values

	Range	Precision		
		Number of Digits	Not Stated	Special Arrangement
1[a]	.588E $\pm$ 38	9		
2	5.6E $\pm$ 76	11		
3	E $\pm$ 99			1–96, by control card (8 if unspecified)
4	E $-$ 46 to E $+$ 69	11		
5	8.758E $-$ 47 to 4.314E $+$ 68		$\checkmark$	
6	5.4E $-$ 79 to 7.2E $+$ 75	7		
7	E $-$ 32 to E $+$ 31	8		
8	.1E $-$ 32 to .99999999E $+$ 31	8		
9	E $\pm$ 308	10		
10	.591E $-$ 39 to 1.694E $+$ 39	7		
11	.687E $\pm$ 308	11		
12	.5E $-$ 308 to .8E $+$ 308	11		
13	E $\pm$ 307	10		
14	E $-$ 293 to E $+$ 322	15		
15	E $-$ 293 to E $+$ 322	15		
16	E $-$ 56 to E $+$ 63	6		
17	E $-$ 56 to E $+$ 63	6		
18	.588E $\pm$ 38	7		
19	E $-$ 32 to E $+$ 30		$\checkmark$	
20	E $\pm$ 99	7		
21	E $\pm$ 75	6		
22	.14E $-$ 38 to 1.7E $+$ 38	8		
23	E $\pm$ 38		$\checkmark$	
24	E $\pm$ 38		$\checkmark$	
25	E $\pm$ 18	8		
26	4.3E $-$ 78 to 5.8E $+$ 76	11		
27	E $\pm$ 76	11		

[a] Compiler number.

TABLE 6 (*continued*)

	Range	Number of Digits	Not Stated	Special Arrangement
		Precision		
28	$E-258$ to $E+254$	9		
29	$E \pm 75$	7		Up to 16, if so written as constants or data
30	$E \pm 38$		√	
31	$E \pm 76$	9		
32	$E \pm 76$	9		
33	$E \pm 127$	8		
34	$E \pm 38$	8		
35	$E \pm 9$		√	
36	$.863616852E-77$ to $.578960444E+77$	9		
37	$E \pm 99$			2–20, by control card
38	$E \pm 76$			6 predecimal, 8 postdecimal
39	Not stated	7		
40	$E \pm 75$	7		
41	$E \pm 75$	7		
42	$E \pm 75$	7		
43	$E \pm 75$	7		
44	$E-39$ to $E+38$	7		
45	$E-100$ to $E+99$			2–20, by control card (8 if unspecified)
46	$E-100$ to $E+99$			1–45, by control card (8 if unspecified)
47	$E-100$ to $E+99$			2–20, by control card (8 if unspecified)
48	$E \pm 99$	8		
49	$E-39$ to $E+38$	7		
50	$E-100$ to $E+99$			3–18, by control card (8 if unspecified)
51	$E \pm 38$	9		
52	$E \pm 38$	9		
53	$E-51$ to $E+49$	8		
54	$E \pm 99$	8		

TABLE 6 (*continued*)

		Precision		
	Range	Number of Digits	Not Stated	Special Arrangement
55	E ± 38	9		
56	5.6E ± 76	11		
57	E ± 115	11		
58	E ± 38	11		
59	E − 150 to E + 147	12		
60	E − 150 to E + 147	12		
61	E ± 616	11		
62	E ± 38	10		
63	E ± 99	12		
64	E ± 75	7		
65	E − 100 to .99999999E + 99	8		
66	E − 100 to .99999999E + 99	8		
67	.432E − 77 to .579E + 77	11		
68	.432E − 77 to .579E + 77	11		
69	1.727E − 77 to 1.236E + 75	6		
70	4.398E − 79 to 7.237E + 75	6		
71	E ± 77	6		
72	E ± 77	11		
73	E ± 38	8		
74	E ± 38	9		
75	E − 50 to E + 49	8		
76	E ± 38	9		
77	E ± 38	9		
78	E − 50 to E + 49	10		
79	No ruling	No ruling		

For Review

hardware
software
exponentiation

Examples

X**4   A**567.

For Review (*continued*)   **Examples** (*continued*)

FORTRAN-supplied functions

$$A = \text{SQRT}(X)$$
$$B = \text{ABS}(C - D)$$
$$E = \text{ALOG}(X) \qquad V = \text{ALOG10}(X)$$
$$F = \text{EXP}(E)$$
$$Z = \text{SIN}(A)$$
$$Y = \text{COS}(A)$$
$$W = \text{ATAN}(Y)$$

argument   Y

subprogram

execution-order rules

exponential notation   3.E+12 ,   4.E−6

normalized number   .3E+13 ,   .4E−5

characteristic   3   ,   4

mantissa   13 ,   −5

range   E ± 99 ,   E ± 38

precision

overflow

underflow

EXERCISES

12. Write a program to find, for $X = 5(10)^9$, square root of X, cube root of X, fourth root of X, fifth root of X, etc.

13. The "compound interest formula"

$$P_n = P_0(1 + r)^n$$

gives the amount of principal (P_n; including accumulated interest) after n periods of investment of P_0 at per period rate r. Write a program to compute and print, for an original principal of \$1000, P_n for the fifth, tenth, fifteenth, twentieth, etc., periods, at interest rate .039.

14. The cosine of an angle X (expressed in radians) may be generated by

$$1 - \frac{X^2}{2!} + \frac{X^4}{4!} - \frac{X^6}{6!} \cdots$$

Write a program that first uses the FORTRAN-supplied function to produce the cosine of 1.14 radians and then forms a loop to generate the series. (As in Exercise 6, you will probably find *two* terms per loop execution a convenient method.)

15. Since the relationship between distance fallen and time falling is

$$d = \tfrac{1}{2}at^2$$

(a = 32.16; see Exercise 3), the elapsed time for fall from any height d must be

$$t = \sqrt{\frac{2d}{a}}$$

Write a program that will produce a table showing the required time for an object to fall 100 feet, 200 feet, 300 feet, etc.

16. The equations governing the dc voltages and currents for the operating point of a transistor stage are:

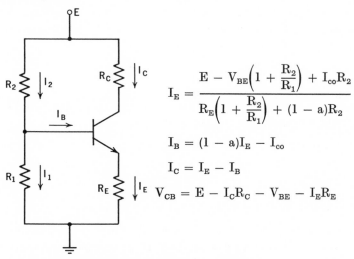

$$I_E = \frac{E - V_{BE}\left(1 + \dfrac{R_2}{R_1}\right) + I_{co}R_2}{R_E\left(1 + \dfrac{R_2}{R_1}\right) + (1 - a)R_2}$$

$$I_B = (1 - a)I_E - I_{co}$$

$$I_C = I_E - I_B$$

$$V_{CB} = E - I_C R_C - V_{BE} - I_E R_E$$

Write a program in which you first define the values

a (current amplification factor)	0.98
V_{BE} (base-to-emitter voltage)	0.30 volts
E (power supply voltage)	12 volts
R_1	10
R_2 (resistances)	33
R_E	1.2 thousand ohms
R_C	2.2

and then compute and print the four quantities defined in the equations, for values of I_{co} (collector leakage current) .005, .010, .015, .020, etc. (milliamperes).

17. Write a program that will produce, for X = 1.001, X^2, X^4, X^8, X^{16}, X^{32}, etc. Try this by more than one method—see if you can discover the shortest possible program.

18. The sum of the squares of the first n natural numbers is given by

$$S = \frac{n(n + 1)(2n + 1)}{6}$$

Write a program that will find S for n = 10, 20, 30, 40, etc.

19. The law of cosines says that

$$a^2 = b^2 + c^2 - 2bc(\cos A)$$

where a, b, and c are the lengths of sides of a triangle and A is the angle opposite a. Write a program to find the length a for a triangle with b = 3 feet and c = 4 feet, for various angles A = 1.39 radians, 1.41 radians, 1.43 radians, etc.

20. The critical level of the correlation coefficient (i.e., a coefficient high enough to provide 99% confidence in correlation within the parent population) may be approximated from

$$r_c = \sqrt{\frac{2.576}{n - 1}}$$

where n is the sample size. Write a program to produce a table showing the critical r for sample size 10, 20, 30, 40, etc.

21. Write a program to evaluate the function

$$\frac{X + 130}{3 \log_e X} + 4X^3$$

for values of X = 1, 2, 3, 4, etc.

22. Since factorial numbers are very large, computer range limitations for storable values are a barrier to computation. (For example, computers with decimal range E ± 38 are limited to 34!, while E ± 76 permits approximately 57!) Therefore, write a program to produce $\log_{10} n!$ for n = 1, 2, 3, 4, 5, etc. (Use a conversion factor to transform the e-base logarithm, if necessary.)

4 · INPUT STATEMENTS— CONDITIONAL BRANCHING— FLOW CHARTS

Input Statements

The programs we have written so far have all been self-contained, in that no data were required during execution; all necessary numerical values were inserted as constants within the source program. In actual practice, such programs are in a small minority, as the phrase "data processing" implies. For the computer is especially valuable where a problem of a particular kind must be handled over and over again, for different data sets. In business, monthly inventory or payroll computations are examples. In statistics, such general methods as correlation analysis or variance analysis may be programmed once for operation on varying data sets. In mathematics, the problem of solving systems of simultaneous equations may be programmed for systems of any size, the size to be specified when a specific problem is executed. In every field, there are recurring problems for which the data may change, but the principles of computation, applicable formulas, and required form of output do not change.

To accommodate the input of data during execution, FORTRAN provides the READ statement:

$$\text{READ (2,100) X, Y, Z}$$

The structure of this statement should be familiar to you, since it parallels the output (WRITE) statement. Thus the first number in parentheses refers to the unit of *input* equipment at which the data will appear, while the second refers to a FORMAT statement, which must specify the precise location and form of the input numbers. The parentheses are followed by an *input list*, which may contain only the names of variables.

Variables mentioned in the input list need *not* have been defined earlier in the program; the READ statement serves to define them. That is, the first

67

input number appearing at input unit number 2 (in the example above) will be stored in the X location, which may or may not have been filled before. If any value *has* previously been in the X location, it will now be replaced by the new input number.

The following program will read punched cards[1] containing employees' wage rates and hours worked and will compute and print their total wages.

```
C       EMPLOYEE WAGES
100     FORMAT (5F15.5)
15    ┌ READ (2,100) RATE, HOURS
      │ WAGES = RATE * HOURS
      │ WRITE (3,100) RATE, HOURS, WAGES
      └ GO TO 15
        END
```

Each execution of the READ statement replaces old values of RATE and HOURS with new ones. (WAGES values are of course replaced each time the *arithmetic* statement is executed.)

Several other forms of the READ statement appear in FORTRAN compilers. For data to be transmitted in internal storage form ("unformatted"— e.g., in binary code), the FORMAT statement reference is omitted:

READ (2) X, Y, Z

For systems with limited input equipment (frequently those for which compiler output statements are PRINT and PUNCH), the equipment unit number is not used. Then the card reader is automatically indicated by

READ 100, X, Y, Z

For input on the typewriter, the statement used may be

ACCEPT 100, X, Y, Z

Input statements that refer specifically to tape units may refer to FORMAT

READ INPUT TAPE 7, 100, X, Y, Z

or be "unformatted"

READ TAPE 7, X, Y, Z

Table 7 shows appropriate forms of the READ statement for various FORTRAN compilers.

---

[1] Presuming that equipment unit number 2 is a card reader.

TABLE 7
Input Statements

(u = equipment unit number; f = FORMAT statement number)

	READ (u,f)	READ (u)	READ f	ACCEPT f	READ INPUT TAPE u,f	READ TAPE u	ACCEPT TAPE f (PAPER TAPE)	READ OTHER
1[a]	✓	✓						
2	✓							
3	✓	✓						
4	✓	✓	✓					
5	✓	✓	✓					
6	✓	✓	✓					
7			✓					INPUT
8			✓		✓	✓		READ FLEX f
9	✓	✓	✓		✓	✓		
10	✓	✓	✓		✓	✓		
11	✓	✓	✓		✓	✓		
12	✓	✓	✓		✓	✓		
13	✓	✓	✓		✓	✓		
14	✓	✓	✓			✓		
15	✓	✓	✓					
16			✓		✓	✓		
17			✓		✓	✓		
18	✓	✓						✓
19								READ f, BUFF
20				✓				READ u, b, f [b = TAPE BLOCK #]
21	✓	✓						
22	✓	✓	✓	✓				
23	✓	✓		✓				
24	✓	✓	✓	✓			✓	
25	✓	✓						
26	✓	✓	✓		✓		✓	
27	✓	✓	✓		✓		✓	

[a] Compiler number.

TABLE 7 (*continued*)

	READ (u,f)	READ (u)	READ f	ACCEPT f	READ INPUT TAPE u,f	READ TAPE u	ACCEPT TAPE f (PAPER TAPE)	READ OTHER
28	✓	✓						READ (u, f, END = #, ERR = #)
29	✓	✓	✓					
30	✓	✓	✓					
31			✓					✓
32	✓		✓		✓	✓		RIPT u, f
33		✓	✓			✓		
34	✓		✓					READ (u) f
35		✓	✓					INPUT
36	✓		✓					✓ INPUT f
37	✓	✓						
38	✓	✓	✓					
39	✓	✓	✓					
40	✓	✓						
41	✓	✓						
42	✓	✓	✓					
43	✓	✓	✓		✓	✓		READ (u, f, END = #, ERR = #)
44	✓	✓	✓		✓	✓		
45			✓		✓	✓		
46	✓		✓		✓			
47	✓	✓	✓		✓	✓		
48			✓	✓			✓	
49	✓							
50	✓	✓	✓					
51	✓	✓						

No.	Statement
52	
53	
54	
55	
56	
57	
58	
59	
60	
61	READ TAPE
62	READ KEYBOARD
63	
64	READ (u, f, END = ✻, ERR = ✻)
65	
66	
67	INPUT (u)
68	INPUT (u)
69	READ (u, f, END = ✻, ERR = ✻)
70	READ (u, f, END = ✻, ERR = ✻)
71	
72	
73	
74	
75	READ (u, f, EOF = ✻)
76	READ INPUT TAPE u
77	
78	
79	

Placement and Form of Data

The data deck for our sample program (containing one card for each employee) is physically completely separate from the source program. It is not used until compilation of the source program has been completed and until the resulting object program has been loaded in core, ready to execute. Any attempt to insert data cards anywhere in the source program would merely provoke compilation error messages, since these cards do not contain translatable FORTRAN statements.

As soon as *execution* of the program has commenced, however, the data deck must be in readiness at the on-line card reader. Each execution of READ causes a card to be passed from the stack to the reading apparatus. If no cards are stacked (or if the reader mechanism has not been properly started up), the execution is halted at the READ instruction. In some systems, this kind of interruption is signaled by explicitly marked console lights (e.g., "READER NO FEED"). In other systems, the reason for the halt is evident only as a particular combination of console display lights. In either case, execution will recommence when the required data have been provided.

For the EMPLOYEE WAGES program, each data card should contain only *numeric* data, since this is all the computer is expecting. The variable *names* (i.e., the names of recipient storage locations) are contained in the *input list*. Any attempt to duplicate them on the data card would lead to execution error (unrecognizable data). That is, the data card should *not* contain

RATE = 4.02   HOURS = 36.

It should say merely

4.02   36.

The FORMAT Statement

Until FORMAT statements are discussed in Chapter 6, we shall use our standard FORMAT for input as well as output. As the sample program illustrates, a single FORMAT statement may be referred to by any number of input and/or output statements.

Since you are already using this standard FORMAT in each of your practice programs, no adjustment is needed to accommodate the input statement. For each exercise requiring data, the sample output in Appendix A is based on a standard data set which is adequately described by

100   FORMAT (5F15.5)

This data set appears at the beginning of the appendix. (Each data card contains five numeric data items, each placed in a 15-column field. Alphabetic data at the right of each card will not be used until Chapter 6.) You should keypunch these data cards (be precise as to column locations) and have them on hand for rapid testing of exercise programs.

Input/Output Unit Control Statements

Most FORTRAN compilers provide three statements (and some provide more) that enable the programmer to manipulate input/output equipment, particularly where tape is the medium being used. In some instances, the statements may be applied to other media as well (e.g., magnetic disk), with comparable results. In the following examples, "u" refers to the appropriate equipment *unit number*.

BACKSPACE u

initiates a backspace of one input record.[2]

REWIND u

causes the specified unit to rewind to its starting point.

END FILE u
or   ENDFILE u

are used to place a mark on the output record that signifies the end of a "file" or data set. (The purpose in most instances is production in later use of a message and/or halt in execution or transfer (branch) to another part of the program, when the end-of-file mark is encountered during input.)

Other unit-control statements occasionally available are

SKIP RECORD u

which initiates a skip of one data record, and

UNLOAD u

which both rewinds and unloads the designated tape unit.

Table 8 shows the availability of these statements in various FORTRAN compilers.

---

[2] "Record" specifies a group of data items being treated as a unit for transmission. The term is formally defined in Chapter 6.

TABLE 8

Input/Output Unit Control Statements

	REWIND u	BACKSPACE u	END FILE u	ENDFILE u	SKIP RECORD u	UNLOAD u	NONE
1[a]	✓	✓		✓			
2				✓			
3	✓	✓		✓			
4	✓	✓	✓				
5	✓	✓		✓			
6	✓	✓	✓				
7							✓
8	✓	✓		✓			
9	✓	✓	✓				
10	✓	✓		✓			
11	✓	✓		✓			
12	✓	✓		✓			
13	✓	✓		✓			
14	✓	✓	✓				
15	✓	✓		✓			
16	✓	✓	✓				
17	✓	✓	✓				
18	✓	✓		✓			
19							✓
20							✓
21	✓	✓	✓				
22	✓	✓	✓		✓	✓	
23	✓	✓		✓			
24	✓	✓		✓			
25							✓
26							✓
27	✓	✓	✓				
28	✓	✓		✓			
29	✓	✓	✓				
30	✓	✓		✓			
31							✓
32	✓	✓	✓				
33	✓	✓	✓				
34	✓	✓	✓				
35							✓
36	✓	✓		✓			
37	✓	✓	✓				
38	✓	✓		✓			
39	✓	✓	✓				

[a] Compiler number.

TABLE 8 (*continued*)

	REWIND u	BACKSPACE u	END FILE u	ENDFILE u	SKIP RECORD u	UNLOAD u	NONE	
40	✓	✓	✓					
41							✓	(Treated as PAUSE u)
42	✓	✓	✓					
43	✓	✓	✓					
44	✓	✓	✓					
45	✓	✓	✓					
46	✓	✓	✓					
47	✓	✓	✓					
48							✓	
49	✓	✓	✓					
50	✓	✓	✓					
51	✓	✓	✓					
52	✓	✓	✓					
53	✓	✓	✓					
54	✓	✓	✓					
55	✓	✓	✓					
56	✓	✓		✓				
57							✓	
58							✓	
59	✓	✓	✓					
60	✓	✓		✓				
61	✓	✓		✓				
62							✓	
63	✓	✓		✓				
64	✓	✓	✓					
65	✓	✓		✓				
66	✓	✓		✓				
67	✓	✓		✓				
68	✓	✓	✓					
69	✓	✓	✓					
70	✓	✓	✓					
71	✓	✓	✓					
72	✓	✓	✓					
73	✓	✓		✓				
74	✓	✓		✓				
75	✓	✓		✓				
76	✓	✓	✓					
77	✓	✓	✓					
78	✓	✓		✓				
79	✓	✓		✓				

A Conditional Branch Statement (The IF Statement)

To this point we have not asked the computer to "make a decision." The phrase is surrounded by quotation marks in recognition of the fact that computers cannot truly make decisions; remember our early statement that the computer will do nothing unless it has been directed explicitly to do it. All "decisions" left to the computer are preplanned by the programmer, who must fully describe all alternative routes and the precise conditions under which each shall be taken. Yet these *conditional branch* arrangements provide tremendous flexibility, permitting large amounts of work with a minimum of human interference during execution.

In the basic conditional branch statement of FORTRAN, the computer is directed to use as a decision criterion the current value of a particular *arithmetic expression*. The expression may consist of a single variable, or any legitimate[3] combination of variables, constants, arithmetic operators, and functions. Three possible results of the expression are distinguished: *negative, zero,* or *positive*.

The form of the statement (beginning in column 7) is:

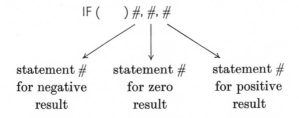

The statement has the effect of three separate GO TO statements. Thus the statement

$$\text{IF (X) 3, 1, 2}$$

may be paraphrased, "If X is negative, GO TO 3; if X is zero, GO TO 1; if X is positive, GO TO 2." In this example, a branch to one of three statements will take place as soon as the current value of X has been looked up in storage.

---

[3] "Legitimate" may be translated as any arithmetic expression ordinarily (in arithmetic statements) acceptable to the compiler. But in some FORTRAN versions, special expressions not usually valid may also appear. These are discussed in Chapters 8 and 10.

More work must be performed prior to branching, when the expression within parentheses contains more than a single variable. Thus

$$\text{IF } (A - B) \ 17, 10, 10$$

is valid, and to the programmer has the interesting meaning, "If A is smaller than B, GO TO 17; if A is equal to or greater than B, GO TO 10." The stored values of A and B are not changed by execution of the statement; this follows the usual rule for variables mentioned in arithmetic expressions (i.e., on the right side of arithmetic statements). Note that *three* statement numbers must be provided, even though one duplicates another.

The IF statement may be used in situations in which the actual purpose is to distinguish between negative, zero, and positive values. For example, the following program reads values of a, b, and c and computes the roots of quadratic equations (general form $ax^2 + bx + c = 0$), using the solution formula

$$\frac{-b \pm \sqrt{b^2 - 4ac}}{2a}$$

```
C        QUADRATIC SOLUTION
100      FORMAT (5F15.5)
4    ┌   READ (2,100) A,B,C
     │   DISCR = B**2 − 4.*A*C
     │   IF (DISCR) 6,5,5
5    │   ROOT1 = (−B−SQRT(DISCR))/(2.*A)
     │   ROOT2 = (−B+SQRT(DISCR))/(2.*A)
     │   WRITE (3,100)A,B,C,ROOT1,ROOT2
     │   GO TO 4
6    │   WRITE (3,100)A,B,C,DISCR
     └   GO TO 4
         END
```

When the discriminant is negative, the roots are imaginary; therefore the program branches around the computation of the roots (which would produce an execution error) and produces as output only a, b, c, and the value of the negative discriminant. Note the necessity of providing for branching *out* (in this case, unconditionally) from each segment of the program entered as an alternative. The omission of the first "GO TO 4" statement would permit entry into a branch of the program not planned by the programmer. Always check arrangements for exit from, as well as entry to, all branches of your programs.

The use of IF for comparison of values in storage is also common technique. The following program reads data items in pairs and reprints only the larger value from each pair. If the values are equal, however, both are printed.

```
C       HIGH VALUES
100     FORMAT (5F15.5)
10   ┌  READ (2,100) ONE, TWO
     │  IF (ONE−TWO) 11,12,13
11   │  WRITE (3,100) TWO
     │  GO TO 10
12   │  WRITE (3,100) ONE, TWO
     │  GO TO 10
13   └  WRITE (3,100) ONE
        GO TO 10
        END
```

Again note the arrangement for branching out from each of the alternative program segments. In connection with this program, be assured that the computer's algebra is perfect. For example, if ONE is −5. and TWO is −7., the positive result of the subtraction identifies ONE as the larger number.

Conditional Limitation of Loops

Another technique using the conditional branch statement is of extreme importance. In each of the programs we have been dealing with, we have created an "endless" loop by using GO TO as a terminal loop statement. We shall now arrange to prelimit the number of executions of statements within a loop. The following program reads exactly 100 data cards, producing as output the products of the two values read from each card. Study it carefully.

```
C       100 PRODUCTS
100     FORMAT (5F15.5)
        COUNT = 0.
54   ┌ READ (2,100) A, B
     │ PROD = A * B
     │ WRITE (3,100) PROD
     │ COUNT = COUNT + 1.
     └ IF (COUNT − 100.)54,66,66
66      STOP
        END
```

STOP, PAUSE, and CALL EXIT Statements

The statement STOP (which may appear anywhere in a program) causes a complete halt to the execution process, returning the computer to control of the operator, rather than leaving it attempting to read a nonexistent data card, as in some of our previous programs. More than one STOP statement may appear in a program (logically, of course, in different *branches* of the program).

While STOP is used for a *terminal* halt, another statement, PAUSE, causes an execution halt that is temporary, since execution recommences with the next executable statement when a console START button is depressed.

To facilitate identification by the programmer of the program branch that has halted the execution, most FORTRAN compilers permit the addition of a (nondecimal) number following the words STOP or PAUSE. This number is reproduced by the computer, when the statement is executed, either as output or by console light display. For example,

PAUSE 66

STOP 30

An important alternative to STOP, in systems under the control of a supervisory program for batch processing,[4] is

CALL EXIT

a statement that returns control to the supervisory program, thus preparing for entry of another job. Table 9 shows applicability to various systems.

TABLE 9

The CALL EXIT Statement

	Available	Not Available
1[a]	√	
2		√
3		√
4		√
5		√
6		√
7		√
8		√
9		√

[a] Compiler number.

---

[4] Stacked entry of many programs and relevant data. (Supervisory systems are discussed in Chapter 12.) In such systems, the use of STOP and PAUSE are not recommended, since the batch-processing concept militates against such interruptions.

TABLE 9 (*continued*)

	Available	Not Available
10		✓
11		✓
12		✓
13		✓
14	✓	
15	✓	
16	✓	
17		✓
18	✓	
19		✓
20		✓
21		✓
22	✓	
23		✓
24		✓
25		✓
26		✓
27	✓	
28		✓
29	✓	
30		✓
31		✓
32		✓
33	✓	
34	✓	
35		✓
36		✓ (BYE or GOODBYE terminates control)
37	✓	
38		✓
39		✓
40	✓	
41	✓	
42		✓
43	✓	
44	✓	
45		✓

TABLE 9 (*continued*)

	Available	Not Available
46		✓
47		✓
48		✓
49	✓	
50	✓	
51	✓	
52	✓	
53		✓
54		✓
55	✓	
56		✓
57	✓	
58	✓	
59		✓
60		✓
61	✓	
62		✓
63	✓	
64	✓	
65		✓
66	✓	
67	✓	
68	✓	
69	✓	
70		✓
71		✓
72		✓
73		✓
74		✓
75		✓
76		✓
77	✓	
78		✓
79		✓

The Loop as the Center of the Program

Our most pressing need for specification (by the programmer) of the number of repetitions to be accomplished in a loop arises in programs that must do further work *after* exit from the loop. For example, the following program reads 50 data items and computes and prints their arithmetic mean (sum of the items, divided by 50):

```
C       MEAN—50 ITEMS
100     FORMAT (5F15.5)
        XNUMB = 0.
        SUMX = 0.
1     ┌ READ(2,100) X
      │ XNUMB = XNUMB + 1.
      │ SUMX = SUMX + X
      └ IF (XNUMB − 50.)1,2,2
2       XMEAN = SUMX/XNUMB
        WRITE (3,100) XMEAN
        CALL EXIT
        END
```

The three-part form of this program is significant, for it is present in the majority of problem-solving programs:

(*a*) Initialization (in this case, one sum and one counter are set to zero).

(*b*) Data input, summation, counting, within a program loop.

(*c*) Terminal computations (employing values computed from the data) and output.

Flow Charting

While we are on the subject of form, we shall look at the process of flow charting, frequently a convenient starting point for complex programs (particularly those employing extensive branching). A flow chart is a schematic diagram of steps that must be executed to solve a problem. Such a chart need *not* contain actual program statements, nor is it necessary to have a separate cell in the flow chart for every program statement that will later be written. If this kind of detail is included, the flow chart becomes a time-waster, rather than an aid in visualizing the program sequence.

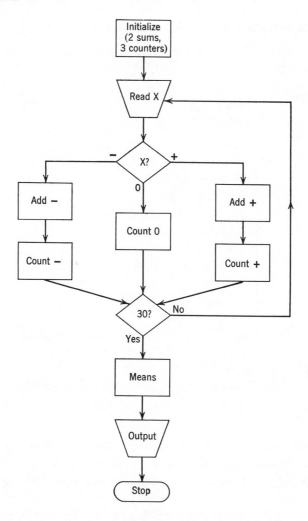

FIG. 11 Flow chart for program producing means of negative and positive data items, and count of zero items.

Let us diagram a program that is to read 30 data items, and compute the mean of the negative items, the mean of the positive items, and the *number* of zero items. The flow chart appears in Fig. 11.

Convention provides different shapes for the cells of the flow chart indicating computation (rectangle), conditional branch (diamond), input/output, and so on.

A program written from the chart follows:

```
C       POSITIVE, NEGATIVE AND ZERO
100     FORMAT (5F15.5)
        SPOS = 0.
        SNEG = 0.
        CPOS = 0.
        CNEG = 0.
        CZERO = 0.
1       READ (2,100) XITEM
        IF (XITEM) 2,3,4
2       SNEG = SNEG + XITEM
        CNEG = CNEG + 1.
        GO TO 5
3       CZERO = CZERO + 1.
        GO TO 5
4       SPOS = SPOS + XITEM
        CPOS = CPOS + 1.
5       IF (CNEG + CPOS + CZERO − 30.)1,6,6
6       XMNEG = SNEG/CNEG
        XMPOS = SPOS/CPOS
        WRITE (3,100) CZERO, XMNEG, XMPOS
        STOP
        END
```

Note that the omission of either "GO TO 5" statement would create a "short circuit" on the flow diagram. But also observe that such a statement is completely unnecessary following the positive-count statement (just prior to statement 5).

We turn now to exercises incorporating the READ and IF statements, for some of which flow charts may be very helpful. Let us first observe, however, that the IF statement is but one form (the most basic) of conditional branch statement. We shall be discussing others shortly. In particular, in the next chapter we look at several other methods of arranging for limitation of repetitive sequences. Therefore, do not adopt the basic IF statement as the only possibility.

For Review	Examples
input statement	READ (2,100) A, B, C
input list	A, B, C

For Review	Examples
input/output control statements	REWIND 7
	BACKSPACE 7
	END FILE 7
	SKIP RECORD 7
	UNLOAD 7
conditional branch statement	IF (A − B) 3, 2, 3
conditional limitation of loops	
execution halt statements	STOP
	STOP 123
	PAUSE
	PAUSE 123
	CALL EXIT
batch processing	
flow chart	

EXERCISES

Note: No more endless loops! In each of the following exercises, limit any program loop by using the IF statement. In many of them, an additional IF statement is required for decisions *within* the loop. For those exercises requiring data, use the standard data set that appears at the beginning of Appendix A (unless special data are listed with the exercise).

23. Write a program that will determine the required size of a round steel bar for each tensile force from 1000 lb to 30,000 lb in increments of 1000 lb. Use the relationships:

$$\text{required area} = \frac{\text{tensile force}}{\text{allowable stress}}$$

$$\text{diameter} = 2\sqrt{\frac{\text{area}}{\pi}}$$

Let allowable stress be 20,000 lb/in.^{2} ($\pi = 3.1415927$). Each output line should include tensile force, required area, and required diameter.

24. A certain microbe culture doubles every hour. Write a program to compute how many microbes will inhabit the culture after 50 hours, starting with one unit. Do it with a loop, with no output until the final result. But also let the program compute and output 2^{50}, using the exponentiation operator, for comparison. Output should all be in *exponential notation*, since the numbers are large (substitute E for F in the standard FORMAT statement).

25. The sum to infinity of the series

$$1 + \frac{1}{2^2} + \frac{1}{3^2} + \frac{1}{4^2} \cdots = \frac{\pi^2}{6}$$

Write a program that shows first as output the expected sum (see Exercise 23 for value of π) and then the sum of the *first 500* terms of the series. Do not output intermediate terms or sums.

26. The *geometric* mean is defined as the nth root of the product of n numbers. The *quadratic* mean is defined as the square root of the mean square of a set of numbers. Write a program to compute and print *both* of these means, for five data items, all keypunched on the same data card.

27. Adjust the program in Exercise 26 so that it will go through the whole read-compute-output process exactly twenty times and test it on the entire data deck.

28. Write a program that reads exactly 15 *pairs* of values (keypunched two per data card) and reprints only those pairs whose sum is greater than 100.0. Also print an identifying number (1.0–15.0) for each pair printed.

29. Write a program that will read exactly 15 data items ("A"—keypunched one per card) and will reprint *only* those that satisfy the following condition:

$$15 \leq A < 20 \quad or \quad A > 40$$

30. Write a program to compute *arithmetic mean* ($\overline{X}$) and *standard deviation* (S_x) of 20 data items, from

$$\overline{X} = \frac{\sum X}{n}$$

and

$$S_x = \sqrt{\frac{\sum X^2}{n} - \overline{X}^2}$$

where n is the number of data items. Note that the numerator term under the radical is a sum of squares, not the square of a sum.

31. Generalize the compound interest program (Exercise 13) by permitting the amount of original principal, and the applicable interest rate, to be read in at execution time. (Test on first two data items.)

32. A thermometer is constructed by employing a thermistor in a Wheatstone bridge. The thermistor is a resistor whose resistance varies with temperature:

$$R_t = R_0 e^{\beta(1/T - 1/T_0)}$$

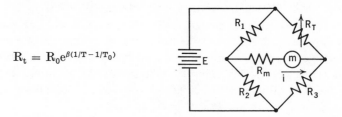

[e = 2.7182818, but a better method is of course EXP(1.)], where R_t is the thermistor resistance at absolute temperature T and R_0 its resistance at absolute temperature T_0. (Absolute temperature = Centigrade temperature + 273.16.)

A bridge is constructed using a thermistor whose β is 3400 and whose resistance R_0 is 1000 ohms when the temperature is 25°C. The other resistors have values R_1 = 2840 ohms, $R_2 = R_3$ = 1000 ohms, R_m = 12,370 ohms and the battery E is 1.500 volts. Prepare a calibration table of meter current i versus temperature for temperatures varying from 0°C to 50°C, in one-degree steps. Use the bridge equation

$$i = \frac{E(R_1 R_3 - R_2 R_T)}{R_m(R_1 + R_2)(R_3 + R_T) + R_1 R_2(R_3 + R_T) + R_3 R_T(R_1 + R_2)}$$

where i is in amperes, E is in volts, and the resistances are in ohms. (The i is rather small, so either switch your FORMAT to exponential notation, as suggested in Exercise 24, or multiply i by 1.E + 6, to convert to microamperes.)

33. A three-period "moving average" for a given series consists of the arithmetic means of the

> 1st, 2nd, and 3rd items,
> 2nd, 3rd, and 4th items,
> 3rd, 4th, and 5th items, etc.

Write a program that will read any number of data items (keypunched *one* per card) and compute and print the three-period moving average, as it reads. (Remember that each READ statement will select a new data card.)

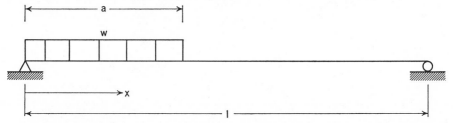

34. A simply supported beam carries a uniform load (w) extending a distance (a) from the left support over a span (l). Write a program that will read w, a, and l and compute and print the *shear* and *moment* at various distances (X) from the left support, from X = 0 to X = 1, in increments of 1/20. Two sets of equations apply:

For $0 \leq X \leq a$	For $a \leq X \leq 1$
$\text{shear} = wa - \dfrac{wa^2}{2l} - wx$	$\text{shear} = -\dfrac{wa^2}{2l}$
$\text{moment} = wax - \dfrac{wa^2 x}{2l} - \dfrac{wx^2}{2}$	$\text{moment} = \dfrac{wa^2}{2} - \dfrac{wa^2 x}{2l}$

35.   According to quantum mechanics, a particle known to be somewhere inside a spherical volume of radius R at some instant t = 0 has a relative probability P of being found at a later time a distance r ≫ R from the center of the sphere, with P being given by

$$P = \left(\frac{r}{a}\right)^{-6}\left(\sin\frac{r}{a} - \frac{r}{a}\cos\frac{r}{a}\right)^2$$

(where a increases linearly with t). Investigate the behavior of this function by computing a table of P versus r/a, letting r/a increase in steps of 0.1, from 0.1 to 2.0.

36.   A 20-card data deck contains two entries per card, representing values for 1960 and 1965 respectively. Write a program that will compute and print:

   (a) Individual ratios, 1965/1960, one per card; but arrange that computation is not attempted where the *1960* value is *zero*.

   (b) The "average" ratio based on the arithmetic mean of those ratios computed in (a).

   (c) The weighted average ratio, based on the 20-item 1960 and 1965 *sums* [which include zero-value lines skipped in (a)].

5 · EXECUTION-TIME OPTIONS—DO STATEMENT— INTEGER VALUES

The Entry of Parameters

We have used the IF statement, in conjunction with a counter, to accomplish limitation of a loop to some predefined number of executions. Our method has been inefficient, in light of our statement that recurrent problems may be programmed once for use on different data sets. For example, in the preceding chapter we wrote a program that computes the arithmetic mean of *fifty* data items. Why not generalize it, to compute the mean of *any number* of data items ? We shall now do so, providing for entry of the parameter[1] n at execution time.

```
C       MEAN — ANY NO. OF ITEMS
100     FORMAT (5F15.5)
        XNUMB = 0.
        SUMX = 0.
        READ (2,100) XN
1       READ (2,100) X
        XNUMB = XNUMB + 1.
        SUMX = SUMX + X
        IF (XNUMB — XN) 1, 2, 2
2       XMEAN = SUMX/XNUMB
        WRITE (3,100) XMEAN
        STOP
        END
```

---

[1] The terminology comes from statistics. A parameter is any characteristic of a population of values. In this instance the relevant parameter is the population's size, symbolized by n.

The changes made include the insertion of a new READ statement (ahead of statement 1) and the replacement of a *constant* by a *variable* in the IF statement. During execution, the data deck must be preceded by a "parameter card" containing the value of n.[2] As an alternative, we could let the operator *type* in the parameter; the first READ statement would then merely specify a different equipment unit number. The generalization of the program that is accomplished in this manner represents good programming technique.

The idea of the parameter card may be extended to the provision of other execution-time options for the operator (or programmer). For example, suppose that in the last program we wanted to provide a choice of either arithmetic *or geometric* mean (nth root of the product of n values). The latter should be computed with logarithms, to avoid the possibility of overflow.

If the arithmetic mean is desired, let the parameter card contain the digit "0" following the n value—while a "1" in this position on the parameter card will indicate geometric mean. The flow chart is drawn in Fig. 12; the program could appear as follows:

```
C       ARITHMETIC OR GEOMETRIC MEAN
C       PARAMETERS—DATA SIZE, FOLLOWED BY
C         0 FOR ARITH., 1 FOR GEOM.
100     FORMAT (5F15.5)
        XNUMB = 0.
        SUMX = 0.
        READ (2,100) XN, TYPEM
1      ⌈READ (2,100) X
       │ IF (TYPEM) 31, 31, 30
30     │ X = ALOG(X)
31     │ XNUMB = XNUMB + 1.
       │ SUMX = SUMX + X
       ⌊ IF (XNUMB − XN) 1, 2, 2
2       XMEAN = SUMX/XN
        IF (TYPEM) 33, 33, 32
32      XMEAN = EXP(XMEAN)
33      WRITE (3,100) XMEAN
        STOP
        END
```

---

[2] Called "XN" in the program, to avoid the IN-letter. Our standard FORMAT requires that this value appear with decimal point keypunched (unless its last digit appears in column 10 of the input data card).

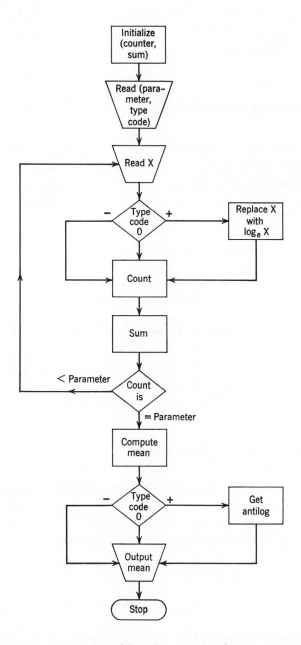

FIG. 12   Flow chart for arithmetic-or-geometric mean program.

The first READ statement has been extended to include the variable signifying required type of mean. Study carefully the arrangements provided by the two added IF statements.

Console Switches for Execution Options

In many systems the computer console is equipped with switches that may be referred to by the programmer as another method of providing options at execution time. The programmer must still write the options into the program, of course. Such "program switches" may be referred to by use of a two-alternative conditional branch statement. Thus

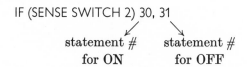

might be used in place of the first IF statement in our choice-of-means program (omitting XN from the first READ statement). Then the operator must put program switch 2 *on* if he wants the geometric mean. This subject is discussed at length in Chapter 8 and is referenced in Table 16.

Limitation of a Loop by Data Termination

In a few systems, the programmer may refer to an *internal* "switch"[3] which provides a method of terminating an input loop without specifying the parameter ("n"). This switch is known as the "last-card indicator." For example, in some compilers written for IBM 1620, the arrangement is

IF (SENSE SWITCH 9) #, #

ON   OFF

The switch referred to is *off* while cards are being read and is turned on by

---

[3] Other "internal switches" are discussed in Chapter 8 and are indexed in Table 17.

passage of the last card through the reader. A mean of data items on cards might then be accomplished as follows:

```
          ----------------
          SUM = 0.
          XNUM = 0.
   1    ┌ READ (2,100) X
        │ SUM = SUM + X
        │ XNUM = XNUM + 1.
        └ IF (SENSE SWITCH 9) 2, 1
   2      XMEAN = SUM/XNUM
          ----------------
```

For most systems a last-card indicator FORTRAN reference statement is not available. However, a simple substitute can be devised by the programmer, which will work on all systems and has the advantage that it will work even though the data are followed by cards representing other jobs. The substitute makes use of a *sentinel card*, a card placed at the bottom of the data deck (behind the last data item). Let this card read, for example, 99999.99, a number known to be outside the range of the data. Then the last sample segment becomes

```
          ----------------
          SUM = 0.
          XNUM = 0.
   1    ┌ READ (2,100) X
        │ IF (X − 99999.99) 11, 2, 2
  11    │ SUM = SUM + X
        │ XNUM = XNUM + 1.
        └ GO TO 1
   2      XMEAN = SUM/XNUM
          ----------------
```

If the data cannot contain *zero* items, the sentinel card may be left *blank*, and the IF statement would be written

$$\text{IF } (X) \ 11, \ 2, \ 11$$

This works because the computer interprets as zero any blank field that corresponds to a variable in an input list.

The DO Statement

The DO statement is an extremely useful shorthand arrangement for specifying the number of repetitions desired in a loop — The following program segment provides for summation of 150 values read from cards:

```
        ----------------------
        SUM = 0.
       ┌DO 14 K = 1, 150
       │READ (2,100) X
   14  └SUM = SUM + X
        ----------------------
```

The total meaning of the DO statement in the sample segment is, "Do everything between here and statement number 14 (inclusive) 150 times."

The general form of the statement is

$$
\#\left[\begin{array}{l} DO \; \# \; K = m_1, m_2, m_3 \end{array}\right.
$$

effect during execution

$$
K = m_1
$$

$$
\left\{\begin{array}{l} K = K + m_3 \\ \qquad\qquad \uparrow\;\uparrow \\ IF \; (K - m_2) \; \#, \#, \# \\ \qquad\qquad\qquad \downarrow \end{array}\right.
$$

where $\#$ is a statement number, which as usual *must* be an *integer* number (no decimal point)

m_1, m_2, m_3 may be *either* integer *constants* or integer *variables*[4] already defined in the program

K must be an integer *variable*, which is defined by the statement (or whose prior value is now replaced by m_1, if it has previously been mentioned in the program)

When the statement is encountered in execution, the following steps are taken:

1. The computer sets up its own counting *index* (K in the sample) and *starts* it at the value m_1.

2. It also provides that, each time statement number $\#$ is executed, the index will be incremented by m_3. If the m_3 position is left blank (omitting the second comma), it is assumed to have the value of 1.

3. After each incrementation, a conditional branch test will be executed. If the incrementation has produced K less than or equal to m_2, the program

---

[4] A full discussion of integer variables and constants appears later in this chapter.

branches *back* to the first executable statement after DO; when the incrementation has produced K greater than m_2, the program branches to the next executable statement following statement number #.[5]

The programmer using the DO statement accomplishes three steps in one,
by comparison with our earlier method of loop control. That is, he initializes a
counter (the DO loop *index*) and arranges at the same time for both its incrementation and the conditional-branch test for its desired limit. As we begin
writing complex programs, it will become evident that a great deal of confusion
is avoided by employing this shorthand looping arrangement. With some exceptions, you should consider using a DO statement whenever any part of your
program is to be repeated.

The general IF statement is not to be discarded, of course. Examine the
following program, which computes the sum of the *larger* members of 200 pairs
of values:

```
C       SUM OF HIGH VALUES
100     FORMAT (5F15.5)
       ⎡SUM = 0.
       ⎢DO 1 NUM = 1,200
       ⎢READ (2,100) X,Y
       ⎢IF (X − Y)2,1,1
2      ⎢X=Y
1      ⎣SUM = SUM + X
        WRITE (3,100) SUM
        STOP
        END
```

Thus the IF statement remains useful, despite our preference for the DO
statement in arranging loops.

Let us review the elements of the DO statement, as illustrated in the last
example.

1. The statement number (1) mentioned after "DO" must refer to an
executable statement (e.g., not FORMAT, COMMENT, END) appearing somewhere *below*, which will be the last one executed before the branch back to the
first executable statement following DO or forward to the next executable
statement after number 1. *No form of branch statement is permitted in this*

---

[5] Thus, subsequent to a normal exit from the loop, the storage situation is $K > m_2$.
In some FORTRAN compilers, however, the conditional test is made before incrementation, leaving $K \leq m_2$ after normal exit. Note that a DO loop is executed *at least once*,
even when $m_1 > m_2$ to begin with (i.e., in the DO statement).

position.[6] Any such statement, conditional or unconditional, would conflict with the branch instruction implicit in the DO statement.

2. NUM (the *index*) is an integer variable, *identifiable as such by the first character of its title:* I, J, K, L, M, or N. This is one of the uses for which we have been reserving the "IN-letters."

3. The starting value of NUM is 1, and its upper limit is 200. The latter is the highest value for which the loop will be executed. The following statement is valid:

DO 5 LOVE = 3,22,2

The increment position is filled in this statement. How many times will statements within the loop (including statement 5) be executed?

LOVE
———

3

5

7

9

11

13

15

17

19

21

The answer is, ten times. Then why not say

DO 5 LOVE = 1,10?

The full answer to this does not become clear until we study subscripted variables (Chapter 7). Then we shall see that the first version might be used to call for selected values of a variable, by utilizing the DO index as a subscript.

Integer Values

In the DO statement use is made of both variables and constants of the *integer* variety. Previously, we have barred their use for ordinary arithmetic statements, with the exception of statement numbers.

An integer *constant* is recognizable by the absence of a decimal point

---

[6] An exception in some compilers is the Logical IF statement, discussed in Chapter 8.

written or punched. An integer *variable* is identified by the use of one of the "IN-letters" as first character of the variable title. In general, integers are used for simple counting purposes (a leading example is the DO statement usage), since (*a*) in such uses, no decimal values need be generated, (*b*) conversely, in ordinary arithmetic decimal values are usually essential. Integers usually require less storage space than decimal values, and operations involving integers are executed more quickly than decimal arithmetic. Therefore, integers *should* be used for counting arrangements.

Two sets of terms have been in use for distinguishing between decimal and integer values. The more recent literature (e.g., manufacturers' manuals) refers to *integer* and *real* constants and/or variables; but in many instances, these are described as *fixed point* (integers) and *floating point* (real) values. The words *fixed* and *floating*, in this context, obviously refer to freedom of the decimal point to appear at various places in the number. For integers, no decimal point appears, and the missing point is therefore assumed to be "fixed" to the right of the last digit. A real value may be written with the decimal point in any position. Exponential notation may be used, in fact, to move the decimal point around without changing the value of the number.

The distinction between these two *modes* is an important one, since the computer treats the integer variable differently from the real variable. Most importantly, the arrangement for *storage* of integer values differs from the usual space allocation. The range of possible values is much smaller for integers than for real values, since integer storage does not provide for exponential representation. For many binary-coded decimal systems, the digital limit is four or five digits, permitting values to plus or minus 9999 or 99999 only. In straight binary systems, the limit is usually $2^n - 1$, in which n represents the number of "bits" allocated for storage of each integer. Table 10 shows the maximum range of integers for various FORTRAN versions.

Table 10 also indicates whether it is permissible to mix integer and real values on the right side of arithmetic statements (i.e., in arithmetic expressions). For all systems, direct combination of real and integer numbers in arithmetic is not possible. In some systems, however, the compiler makes provision for temporary conversion (*floating*) of integer values appearing in such *mixed expressions* (e.g., changing 124 to .124E + 3), for the purpose of computation. Therefore

$$XMEAN = SUM/N$$

or $\quad X = X + 1$

or $\quad J = W * M$

TABLE 10

Integer Values

	Range		Mixed Expressions, Real and Integer			Explicit Type Specification Real and Integer	
	$2**N-1$	Plus or Minus	Allowed	Not Stated	Error	Available	Not Available
1[a]	29	536 870 911			✓		✓
2	23	8 388 607			✓	✓	
3	[1–99 digits, by control card—if unspecified, 99 999]				✓	✓	
4	39	549 755 813 887		✓		✓	
5	39	549 755 813 887	✓			✓	
6	31	2 147 483 647	✓			✓	
7	11	2 047	✓				✓
8	22	4 194 303	✓				✓
9	47	140 737 488 355 327	✓			✓ (preceded by TYPE)	
10	15	32 767			✓	✓	
11	23	8 388 607	✓			✓	
12	23	8 388 607	✓			✓	
13	47	140 737 488 355 327	✓			✓	
14	59	576 460 752 303 423 487	✓			✓	
15	59	576 460 752 303 423 487	✓			✓	
16	22	4 194 303	✓				✓
17	[All arithmetic in real; $E-56$ to $E+63$]		✓				✓
18	15	32 767			✓		✓
19	[$10^4 - 1$]	9 999			✓		✓
20	11	2 047			✓		✓
21	17	131 071			✓	✓	
22	35	34 359 738 367	✓			✓	
23	15	32 767			✓	✓	
24	15	32 767			✓	✓	
25	17	131 071	✓				✓
26	23	8 388 607	✓				✓
27	23	8 388 607	✓			✓	

[a] Compiler number.

TABLE 10 (*continued*)

	Range		Mixed Expressions, Real and Integer			Explicit Type Specification Real and Integer	
	2 ** N − 1	Plus or Minus	Allowed	Not Stated	Error	Available	Not Available
28	$[10^{11} - 1]$	99 999 999 999	✓				✓
29	31	2 147 483 647	✓			✓	
30	39	549 755 813 887			✓		✓
31	19	524 287	✓				✓
32	19	524 287			✓	✓	
33	23	8 388 607			✓	✓	
34	35	34 359 738 367			✓	✓	
35	23	8 388 607	✓			✓	
36	19	524 287	✓			✓	
37	17 to 71	[By control card]			✓	✓	
38	23	8 388 607			✓	✓	
39	Not stated	"7 digits"	✓			✓	
40	31	2 147 483 647	✓			✓	
41	31	2 147 483 647			✓		✓
42	31	2 147 483 647	✓			✓ [b]	
43	31	2 147 483 647	✓			✓	
44	15	32 767	✓			✓	
45	[1–20 digits, by control card— if unspecified, 99 999]				✓		✓
46	[1–99 digits, by control card— if unspecified, 99 999]				✓		✓
47	[1–20 digits, by control card— if unspecified, 99 999]				✓	✓	
48	$[10^4 - 1]$	9 999			✓		✓
49	15	32 767	✓			✓	
50	[3–20 digits, by control card— if unspecified, 99 999]				✓	✓	
51	35	34 359 738 367			✓		✓
52	35	34 359 738 367			✓	✓	
53	$[10^{10} - 1]$	9 999 999 999			✓		✓
54	$[10^{10} - 1]$	9 999 999 999			✓		✓

[b] Also performs functions of DATA statement.

TABLE 10 (*continued*)

	Range		Mixed Expressions, Real and Integer			Explicit Type Specification Real and Integer	
	$2 ** N - 1$	Plus or Minus	Allowed	Not Stated	Error	Available	Not Available
55	35	34 359 738 367			✓	✓	
56	23	8 388 607	✓			✓	
57	36	68 719 476 733	✓			✓	
58	47	140 737 488 355 327	✓			✓	
59	$\begin{bmatrix} -10^{11} - 1 \\ +10^{12} - 1 \end{bmatrix}$	− 99 999 999 999 to +999 999 999 999	✓				✓
60	$\begin{bmatrix} -10^{11} - 1 \\ +10^{12} - 1 \end{bmatrix}$	− 99 999 999 999 to +999 999 999 999	✓			✓	
61	39	549 755 813 887			✓	✓	
62	21	2 097 151			✓		✓
63	23	8 388 607			✓	✓	
64	31	2 147 483 647	✓			✓	
65	$[10^7 - 1]$	9 999 999			✓		✓
66	$[10^7 - 1]$	9 999 999			✓	✓	
67	23	8 388 607			✓		✓
68	23	8 388 607	✓			✓	
69	31	2 147 483 647	✓			✓	
70	31	2 147 483 647	✓			✓	
71	15	32 767			✓	✓	
72	23	8 388 607			✓	✓	
73	17	131 071			✓	✓	
74	29	536 870 911	✓			✓	
75	$[10^5 - 1]$	99 999			✓	✓	
76	35	34 359 738 367	✓			✓	
77	35	34 359 738 367	✓			✓	
78	$[10^6 - 1]$	999 999			✓	✓	
79	No ruling		No ruling			✓	

are valid statements in such systems. In other systems, however, such statements would draw a compilation error message, "*mixed mode*," and compilation could not be completed until the programmer made suitable changes.

This mixing prohibition refers only to the *right* side of arithmetic statements (hence to expressions within parentheses of IF statements). The following statements are valid in *all* systems:

$$X = J + 1$$
$$K = 10.2/SUM$$

The *result* of such statements must be carefully noted, however. If $J = 3$ when the first is executed, X is stored as .4E + 1, a real value. In the second statement, if SUM = 2.0, the result 5.1 cannot be stored in location "K" except as "5." This sort of truncation will be discussed further in the next section.

Another exception to the "mixed mode" rule was noted in Chapter 3: *exponents* may be in integer mode, even though their arguments are real.

Integer Arithmetic

Arithmetic using integers exclusively is possible in all systems. Thus

$$K = K + 1$$
$$\text{or} \quad MONEY = ITEMS * KASH$$

are perfectly valid statements.

Since the spelling seems a bit peculiar in the last instance, let us digress to mention a possibility available in most compilers. The programmer may employ *explicit type specification*, by using a nonexecutable statement(s) to indicate that certain variables are to be treated as though they are of opposite mode from what the *implicit* specification of their first title-character suggests. Thus

$$\text{INTEGER CASH, FUNDS}$$
$$\text{REAL LUCK, JOB, NEWS}$$

are nonexecutable[7] statements that will be used during compilation to reserve appropriate storage for the variables named. Such statements must appear in the program ahead of any executable statements. Following the sample statements,

$$MONEY = ITEMS * CASH$$

---

[7] Other nonexecutable statements are discussed in Chapters 6 (FORMAT), 7 (DIMENSION), 9 (FUNCTION, SUBROUTINE, COMMON, EXTERNAL), 10 (DOUBLE PRECISION, COMPLEX, LOGICAL), 11 (IMPLICIT, EQUIVALENCE, DATA), and 12 (DEFINE FILE).

would be executed entirely in integer mode, since "CASH" values would have been stored as integers and be so treated throughout the program. In the absence of the explicit type declaration, ITEMS would have been *floated*, and the arithmetic performed in real mode, *or* an error would have resulted, in systems not permitting mixed expressions. Note that following the two specification statements shown,

$$DO\ 5\ JOB = 1,\ 175$$

would be invalid, while

$$DO\ 5\ FUNDS = 1,175$$

would be acceptable.

Table 10 indicates availability of the REAL and INTEGER declarations, in various FORTRAN compilers.

The use of integers in arithmetic must be approached with caution by the programmer. We have already mentioned the problem of *truncation* in integer *division*. The result of

$$J = 27/4$$
$$is\quad J = 6$$

Similarly, the result of

$$X = 27/4$$
$$is\quad X = 6.0$$

Thus the programmer who expects decimal results will be disappointed. This truncation occasionally may be used, however, as the basis for tricks in programming. For example, the following statement will distinguish between *odd* and *even* values of K (branching to statement 6 for even and to 7 for odd):

$$IF\ (K/2 * 2 - K)\ 7,\ 6,\ 7$$

The truncation takes place instantly when the division is performed, so that K = 31 produces

$$IF\ (30 - 31)7,6,7$$

while K = 32 would produce

$$IF\ (32 - 32)7,6,7$$

The technique obviously may be generalized to determine divisibility (factorability) by any integer value.

The freedom to write a different mode on the *left* side of an arithmetic statement as compared to the (consistent) *right*-side mode also makes possible some tricks. The following segment distinguishes between X values that are integers[8] (branch to 9) and those that are not (branch to 8):

$$L = X$$
$$W = L$$
$$IF\ (W - X)8,9,8$$

Another reason for caution in using integers for arithmetic is the much lower maximum storable value. If K = 123456,

$$M = K * K$$

produces nothing but trouble, since the result cannot be stored in an integer location, in most systems. Nor will

$$G = K * K$$

be any better, since the *overflow* takes place as soon as the multiplication is attempted.

Integer variables may be mentioned in input and/or output lists. However, our standard FORMAT statement is designed to accommodate only real variables. In the next chapter we shall acquire the necessary flexibility.

Variable Input/Output Unit Specification

The equipment unit number mentioned in each input and output statement may be presented as an *integer variable*, instead of an integer constant. This permits treatment of the choice of input or output equipment as an execution-time option. For example, a parameter card may be utilized:

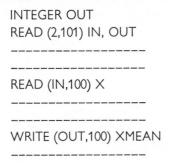

```
INTEGER OUT
READ (2,101) IN, OUT
------------------
------------------
READ (IN,100) X
------------------
------------------
WRITE (OUT,100) XMEAN
------------------
```

[8] That is, they have only zero content to the right of the decimal point. The X is, of course, in real, not integer, mode.

In this example, FORMAT 101 must contain the proper specifications for an integer variable. Note that a FORMAT statement number may *not* be anything but an integer constant.

The CONTINUE Statement

The statement CONTINUE, found in all FORTRAN versions, is translated to a machine language statement signifying "no operation." There is only one legitimate use for such a statement, and that is as the last statement of a DO loop. When so used, it is there because the programmer wishes to branch to the end of the loop *in order to preserve the count by incrementing and testing the DO index.* For example, the following program reads 50 values and computes the sum for only those that are integers.

```
C       INTEGERS
100     FORMAT (5F15.5)
        SUM = 0
       ┌DO 2 I = 1,50
       │READ (2,100) X
       │K = X
       │G = K
       │IF (G − X)2,1,2
1      │SUM = SUM + X
2      └CONTINUE
        WRITE (3,100) SUM
        END
```

Remember that the proper way to get to the *top* of a DO loop is to branch to the *bottom*. If the programmer branched from the IF statement straight back to the READ statement, the sample program would not produce any output. Be sure that you understand why.

Optional Data Size with DO Loops

To generalize a program that uses one or more DO statements, the parameter-entry and the data-termination methods are both usable. For the former, a combination of statements such as

```
READ (2,101) N
DO 4 K = 1,N
```

will accomplish the desired result. FORMAT 101 must contain proper notation for an integer variable. As an alternative, our standard FORMAT could be used as follows:

```
READ (2,100) RN
N = RN
DO 4 K = 1,N
```

In fact, conversion of the parameter n to real mode is frequently necessary when it has been read in as an integer, since it may be needed for "real" arithmetic—for instance, as divisor for computation of the data mean.

The last-card method (e.g., using a sentinel card) may be implemented by "jumping" out of a DO loop with a conditional branch statement. Thus

```
C       MEAN—UP TO 5000 DATA ITEMS
100     FORMAT (5F15.5)
        SUM = 0.
      ┌ DO 3 N = 1,5000
      │ READ (2,100) X
      │ IF (X − 99999.)3,4,4
3     └ SUM = SUM + X
4       XNUM = N − 1
        XMEAN = SUM/XNUM
        WRITE (3,100) XMEAN
        STOP
        END
```

The program works for any number of data items up to 5000. Notice the single-statement adjustment and conversion that produce the parameter in real mode.

In review of some of our recently acquired techniques, let us construct a program to read n values and select and print the smallest.

A sound approach to any programming problem is to ask, "How would the problem be solved *without* a computer? How would you, for example, select the smallest value from any set of values? Your ability to break the process down into separate sequential steps is the prerequisite for programming it. The usual method would be described something like this:

1. Examine the first value. Remember it (it is the smallest, so far.)

2. Examine the next value; if it is larger than the one you remember, ignore it and examine the third. If it is smaller, however, remember it instead of the other.

3. Examine the next value, etc.

4. When all values have been examined, the one "remembered" is the smallest.

A translation to computer programming terms might read:

1. *Read* a value.

2. *Read* another; *compare* this and the other. If this is larger, *continue*. If this is smaller, *replace* the other.

3. *Repeat* the read/compare/continue-or-replace sequence until data are exhausted.

4. *Output* the stored value.

The required program statements are suggested by consultation with our accumulated FORTRAN glossary:

English	FORTRAN
read	READ
repeat	DO
compare	IF
replace	=
continue	CONTINUE
output	WRITE

We shall read n (number of data items) from a parameter card. The program appears as follows:

```
C       SMALLEST VALUE
100     FORMAT (5F15.5)
        READ (2,100) XNUM
        READ (2,100) SMALL
        NUM = XNUM
       ┌DO 2 K = 2, NUM
       │READ (2,100) X
       │IF (X − SMALL) 1, 2, 2
1      │SMALL = X
2      └CONTINUE
        WRITE (3,100) SMALL
        CALL EXIT
        END
```

Nested DO Loops

Frequently it is convenient to have two or more DO loops operating simultaneously in a program. For example, the following program is designed to accomplish 10 separate sums, each utilizing 50 items of a 500-card data deck:

```
C       TEN SUMS, FIFTY ITEMS EACH
100     FORMAT (5F15.5)
        ┌DO 2 I = 1, 10
        │SUM = 0.
        │┌DO 1 J = 1, 50
        ││READ (2,100) X
1       ││SUM = SUM + X
2       └WRITE (3,100) SUM
        CALL EXIT
        END
```

Note that each loop requires a separate *index*. In this example certain statements (the sum initialization and the output statement) are executed as part of the outer loop, but form no part of the inner loop. Any statements in the inner loop (e.g., the READ statement) are executed m × n times, where m and n are the respective numbers of specified executions for each loop.

It is permissible to have two or more DO loops end at the same statement. In such cases, the computer, faced with more than one increment-test-branch chore each time this statement is reached, gives precedence to the *innermost* loop—that is, to the DO statement most recently encountered. For example,

```
C       COMBINATIONS
        ┌DO 1 L = 1, 4
        │J = L + 1
        │┌DO 1 K = J, 5
1       └└WRITE (3,101) L, K
```

The program segment prints all possible *combinations* of the numbers 1 through 5. The inner-loop precedence rule indicates that the output will be as follows:

1	2
1	3
1	4
1	5
2	3
2	4
2	5
3	4
3	5
4	5

Overlapping DO loops are not permitted. That is, the segment

```
       --------------
      ┌DO 12 I = 1, 10
      │READ (2,100) X
      │┌DO 13 J = 1, 15
  12  └│A = 14. * X**2
  13   └WRITE (3,100) A
       --------------
```

is illegal.

For Review	Examples
execution-time option	
parameter card	
console switches	IF (SENSE SWITCH 2) 3, 4
last-card indicator	IF (SENSE SWITCH 9) 5, 6
sentinel card	IF (X − 9.E+20) 3, 4, 3
DO statement	DO 13 K = 1, 100
	DO 15 LUMP = J, K, L
DO loop index	LUMP
integer variable	K, ITEM
integer constant	65, 99999
real variable	A, BAKER
real constant	3.2, .32E+1
fixed point	(= integer)
floating point	(= real)
mode	
mixed mode	A = B + I
explicit type specification	REAL K, JOHN
	INTEGER B, CODE, V
implicit type specification	
truncation	
variable I/O unit specification	
CONTINUE statement	5 CONTINUE
nested DO loops	

EXERCISES

Note: From this point on, you should normally be using the DO statement to arrange program loops, reserving the IF statement for other decisions.

37. Write a program that will read two data items at a time, and print them in ascending size order. The program should then go back and read another pair of values, etc. In all, 20 pairs should be read, arranged, and printed.

38. A payroll system uses one card for each employee, on which appear (*a*) hourly wage rate and (*b*) number of hours worked during the month. Write a program that utilizes a *sentinel card* to read all the data and compute and print (1) total wage bill for the month and (2) arithmetic mean and standard deviation of the wage rates. (See Exercise 30 for formulas.)

39. Write a program to print a table of X, $\log_e$ X, and sine X for X values of 1.0, 1.1, 1.2, up to and including 2.0, and then stop. Can this be done *without* defining X outside of the program's main loop?

40. The sum to infinity of the series

$$1 - \tfrac{1}{2} + \tfrac{1}{3} - \tfrac{1}{4} + \tfrac{1}{5} \cdots$$

is $\log_e$ 2. Write a program that finds the sum of the first 1000 terms, and also prints $\log_e$ 2, for comparison. Output must be limited to these two values.

41. The National Board of Fire Underwriters stipulates that the total fire-stream capacity to be provided in the design of a municipal water distribution system shall be

$$Q = 1012\sqrt{P}\left(1 - \frac{\sqrt{P}}{100}\right)$$

where Q = rate of flow in qpm
      P = population, in thousands
Write a program that will compute Q for populations ranging from 1000 to 9000 by increments of 1000; from 10,000 to 90,000 by increments of 10,000; and from 100,000 to 900,000 by increments of 100,000. Use a double DO loop in your program.

42. Write a program to read 20 values of X and W (keypunched in that order, two data items per card) and compute and print the unweighted arithmetic mean *and* the weighted mean

$$\overline{X} = \frac{\sum X}{n} \qquad \overline{X}_w = \frac{\sum wX}{\sum w}$$

43. The sum to infinity of

$$1 + \frac{1}{1!} + \frac{1}{2!} + \frac{1}{3!} \cdots$$

is equal to e, the base of the natural logarithm system. Write a program that computes this sum through 1/20! Produce as output only the final result (not intermediate sums). Also devise a method of producing the actual value e as output for comparison (*without* reading it in as data or inserting it as a constant in the source program).

44. Write a program that will read 20 data items (one per card) and compute and print $\log_e$ n! for *each* of the 20 values (or for the next lowest integer, in the case of noninteger values). Use two DO loops.

45. Write a program that will number 15 lines,

$$1.00000$$
$$2.00000$$
$$3.00000$$
$$1.00000$$
$$2.00000$$
$$3.00000$$
$$1.00000$$
$$\text{etc.}$$

46. Write a program that will read 20 real values, and reprint only those that are *odd integers*.

47. Write a program to produce n and cube root of n for n = 50, 55, 60, . . . , 100 and then stop.

48. Write a program that will read 20 real values, and reprint only the *postdecimal* portion of each.

49. The "t" test generates a statistic with predictable distribution, which is based on the difference between any two sample means. It may be computed from

$$t = \frac{\overline{X}_a - \overline{X}_b}{\hat{\sigma}_d}$$

in which $\hat{\sigma}_d$ is obtained from

$$\hat{\sigma}_d = \sqrt{\frac{\hat{\sigma}_x{}^2}{n_a} + \frac{\hat{\sigma}_x{}^2}{n_b}}$$

which in turn makes use of

$$\hat{\sigma}_x{}^2 = \frac{\sum X_a{}^2 - n_a\overline{X}_a{}^2 + \sum X_b{}^2 - n_b\overline{X}_b{}^2}{n_a + n_b - 2}$$

Write a program that will compute t, for input data consisting of:

(*a*) ten values of X_a, keypunched one per card and
(*b*) ten values of X_b, keypunched one per card.

Let output include both means, the estimated population variance ($\hat{\sigma}_x{}^2$), the estimated standard error ($\hat{\sigma}_d$), and t.

6 · FORMAT
STATEMENTS

The transfer of information between core storage and input/output media is usually accomplished, as we have seen, by a combination of input or output statement and FORMAT statement. The I/O statement specifies the equipment to be used and lists the variables to be transmitted (i.e., names the core storage locations in which input data will be stored or from which output values will be copied). The function of the FORMAT statement is description of the precise *form* and *position* of data.

We begin by defining some of the terms used in the following discussion.

A *field* is any set of characters (columns) to be treated as a unit for transmission, storage, and so on. We shall refer to the field as being "w" characters in width.

A *record* is a set of fields treated as a unit during transfer of information. For punched cards, each card is considered a separate record. Thus a card record may have eight ten-column fields, or twenty four-column fields, and so on. For other media (tape, disk, etc.) record length is indicated by special "end-of-record" marks, inserted as the initial inscription is performed.

Numeric fields contain only numeric information (which may include, in addition to numeric digits, decimal points, plus and minus signs, and the E that precedes exponent information).[1]

Alphameric fields may contain *any* combination of characters that may be keypunched, including alphabetic and special characters as well as digits.

Figure 13 lists basic characters[2] that may appear within a FORMAT statement.

---

[1] A "D" that performs the same function for double precision values is discussed in Chapter 10.

[2] Some additional characters will be discussed in Chapter 11 (listed in Table 26).

F Notation, Output

Our standard FORMAT statement

100   FORMAT (5F15.5)

actually says, "five variables, real (decimal) notation, in fields of fifteen characters, each with five decimal places." The general form of such specifications is

nFw.d

in which "n" may be used to repeat the specification and "d" indicates post-decimal length of the field. The "n" (if it appears), "w", and "d" must all be integer constants. If "n" is omitted, a value of "1" is assumed. Thus

F12.2

specifies ordinary decimal notation for a single real variable. Total field width is twelve characters, the last three of which are to be decimal-point and two postdecimal digits.

Numeric fields

F	Real data, decimal form
I	Integer data
E	Real data, exponential form

Positional

X	Blank column
/	New record

Alphameric fields

H	Transfer (of following characters) between I/O medium and FORMAT statement
' '	Transfer (of enclosed characters) between I/O medium and FORMAT statement
A	Transfer between I/O medium and labeled storage

Separation

,	Separates notation items (where necessary for clarity)
.	Separates field width ("w") and decimal-field width ("d") instructions.

FIG. 13   FORMAT notation characters.

The computer will *right-justify* numeric output within the specified field width (producing blanks at the left of the field) and will *truncate* (without rounding) digits to the right of the postdecimal position specified for output. Thus the value in storage 1234.5678 will be reproduced in F12.2 as

bbbbb1234.56

(b indicating blank column).

A change in "w" alters the horizontal position of output. Thus F9.2 would produce

bb1234.56

A change in "d" alters the postdecimal content. Thus F9.3 produces

b1234.567

A notation specification should be provided for each variable appearing in the output list. For example,

WRITE (3,10) A, B, C, D, E

10   FORMAT (3F10.4,F5.0,F6.2)

Variables A, B, and C are produced in F10.4, while D and E receive different treatment. Forty-one total characters constitute the output record. (Note that the F5.0 field ends with a decimal point.) The comma used for separation of instructions can usually be dispensed with, unless its absence would make the meaning of *consecutive digits* ambiguous. For example,

(F10.3,2F6.1)

cannot be written without the comma.

If the output list has fewer variables than the number of specifications contained in FORMAT, extra specifications are simply ignored. (For example, our standard FORMAT statement is capable of outputting five *or fewer* variables.) If the output list is *longer* than the number of specifications provided, the FORMAT statement is reused, starting from the nearest left parenthesis. Thus

WRITE (3,11) A, B, C. D, E

11   FORMAT (F10.1, F5.0)

will be the equivalent of

11   FORMAT (F10.1,F5.0,F10.1,F5.0,F10.1)

Repetition of a *group* of specifications may be called for by placing the group in parentheses and indicating the number of repetitions with an integer constant ahead of the left parenthesis. For example,

$$\text{WRITE (3,12) NUM, X, L, Y, M, Z, N}$$
$$\text{12   FORMAT (I10,3(F10.2,I5))}$$

produces all output as though written

$$\text{12   FORMAT (I10,F10.2,I5,F10.2,I5,F10.2,I5)}$$

Determination of appropriate size for "w" and "d" is dependent on several considerations:

1. The "count" begins at the left (column 1) of each new record; but the second specification describes a field beginning at the right end of the first, the third field begins at the right end of the second, and so on. Thus

$$\text{(F10.2,F20.2)}$$

occupies 30 total columns, not 20.

2. As "w" increases, the output value is moved to the right. Left-hand characters in the field remain blank. For example,

(F5.1)	12.3
(F8.1)	12.3

3. As "d" increases, the number of postdecimal digits in output is increased. The right-justified output position does not change, but some left-hand blanks are replaced by predecimal digits. For example,

(F8.1)	12.3
(F8.3)	12.345

4. Large values of "d" produce nonsignificant digits at the right of the field, but do not produce error. Small "d" values produce truncation of postdecimal digits, but do not produce error. The minimum "d" value is zero, which must be keypunched. For example,

(F12.8)	12.34567800
(F12.0)	12.

5. Overly small "w" specifications lead to *execution* errors, when data values to be output are too large for the specified field. For example,

(F3.1)   cannot output the stored value 12.345678

The total field specified must be wide enough to hold in all systems:

the number of postdecimal digits mentioned in "d"
the actual number of predecimal digits contained in the output value
the decimal point
a minus sign, if the output value is negative

In some systems, additionally it must hold:

a space for the sign, even if it is positive and therefore not printed
a space for a predecimal zero, in the absence of predecimal content

Thus a "stingy" specification such as

$$(\text{F4.1})$$

could successfully output, in all systems, a number such as 1.2345678:

$$b1.2$$

However, the number 12.345678 would produce execution error in some systems (no room for sign), and -12.345678, or 123.45678, would cause error in all systems. Similarly,

$$(\text{F3.1})$$

could not be used to reproduce the value $-.12345678$ in systems that print a leading predecimal zero.

    6. As a corollary of the rules outlined in (5), the relationship *between* "w" and "d" that is acceptable in all systems is

$$w \geq d + 3$$

since this leaves room for the decimal point, sign, and at least one predecimal digit. Thus

$$\text{F4.1, F5.2, F6.3, etc.}$$

meet minimal w-to-d requirements. We have already noted, however, that their success during *execution* depends on the size of output values encountered. Systematic planning to avoid execution error will be discussed at the end of this chapter.

F Notation, Input

Our standard FORMAT statement, when referenced by an *input* statement, describes an input record consisting of five 15-character fields, each containing a data item in real form, that is, with decimal point. If a decimal point actually does appear in the input field, *its position takes precedence over the "d" part of the FORMAT specification.* Furthermore, this rule permits the data item key-punched with decimal point to appear anywhere in the field; it need not be right-justified. Thus if an input field contains

12.345678bbbb

the data value read in F13.4 is stored as 12.3456. If no decimal point appears in the input field, then the FORMAT "d" value supplies its position, and right-justification in the input field becomes important. Thus a field containing

bbbbb12345678

will be stored (if read in F13.4) as 1234.5678. If it were placed in the input field as

12345678bbbbb

the value stored would be 123456780.0000 (represented internally, of course, as .12345678 + 09).

If the input list has fewer variables than the number of specifications in FORMAT, extra specifications are ignored (as in output). Thus our standard FORMAT statement reads five *or fewer* data items from a single record. If, however, the number of FORMAT specifications is too few for the list appearing in the input statement, *the reuse of FORMAT from the left parenthesis causes selection of a new record.* Therefore

READ (2,10) A, B, C, D, E, F
10   FORMAT (F10.2)

has the effect of reading a single value from each of six separate records (e.g., six successive punched cards). We may note that this is the same effect as would be obtained from

10   FORMAT (F10.2/F10.2/F10.2/F10.2/F10.2/F10.2)

in which the slash (discussed below) indicates "new record."

It must also be remembered that each execution of a READ statement automatically selects a *new* record. Thus the use of six separate records results from

```
        ┌DO 1 I = 1,6
        │READ (2,15) X
        │------------
        │------------
    1   └------------
   15    FORMAT (10F6.1)
```

Nine "extra" specifications are ignored, at each execution of the READ statement.

I Notation, Output

The general notation form for integer data is

$$nIw$$

As usual, "n" may be omitted, in which case it has an assumed value of "1." The output value is right-justified in the specified field and will be moved to the right by increasing the value of "w." Thus the value 1234 will appear in I7 as

bbb1234

and in I5 as

b1234

Execution error may result from overly narrow "w" size. Thus the value 123456 cannot be handled in I5. The minimum value of "w" acceptable in compilation is "2" for systems that reserve room for the sign and "1" for others.

I Notation, Input

Right-justification of input data in the specified field is extremely important, since blanks to the right of actual digits will be interpreted as zeros. Thus

bbb123bbb

will be interpreted by I9 as 123000. If 123 is to be stored, I6 is correct.

From the discussion so far, it should be clear that a continuous string of digits appearing on an input record may be interpreted as separate data items. For the data

123456789

the following statements

READ (2,16) I, A, J, B

16   FORMAT (I2,F2.0,I3,F2.1)

produce

I = 12
A = 34.0
J = 567
B = 8.9

E Notation, Output

The general specification form for data in exponential notation is

nEw.d

The programmer's use of exponential notation for output is normally predicated on his expectation of very large or very small real values. For example, we have indicated that execution error would result from attempting to print the stored value 123456780000.0 in such F notation as F13.4. If instead we specify E13.4, we obtain, in some systems,

1234.5678E+08

We may observe that the value of "d" is immaterial, in the sense that the exponent and decimal point change in opposite directions when "d" changes. For example, E13.7 for this value produces, in the same systems,

1.2345678E+11

For this reason, many compilers standardize exponential output by always producing it in what was described in Chapter 3 as the "normalized" form. That is, the decimal point is placed at the left of the output field (except for a leading zero), and to its right are printed only the "d" leftmost digits of the stored value. Thus E13.4 would produce (for our sample value)

0.1234E+12

and E13.7 would give

0.1234567E+12

This suggests that a good method of handling E notation for output, for effective compatibility with all systems, is to *make "d" equal to the computer's precision limit for real values* (see Table 6).

For small values, E notation produces significant digits, when F notation may produce many nonsignificant zeros. For example, for the stored value .00000012345678, F16.8 produces

$$.00000012$$

whereas E16.8 produces

$$0.12345678E-06$$

The relationship between "w" and "d" that is acceptable in all systems is

$$w \geq d + 7$$

which leaves room for the four characters of E notation, decimal point, sign, and at least one predecimal digit (a leading zero, in many systems).

E Notation, Input

Input data that are referred to by E specifications in FORMAT may appear in several forms. When an exponent appears, the entire value should be right-justified in the input field. Each of the following is valid:

$$1.E + 09$$
$$1.E + 9$$
$$1.E9$$
$$1E9$$

Since decimal points in the input record have precedence as usual, the first three examples will be stored as the real number 1000000000.0 (internal form .1E + 10), regardless of the size of "d" in the E specification appearing in FORMAT. In the fourth example, however, the FORMAT specification will control the decimal-point location. Therefore

$$E10.0$$

would result in the interpretation .1E + 10, whereas

$$E10.4$$

would produce

$$.1E + 06.$$

If reference to the exponent is omitted from the input data field, the exponent is presumed to be zero. Thus any real value (punched with decimal point) may be read by any E specification. Right-justification in the input field is not necessary. For example,

12.34

will be interpreted as 12.34 by Ew.d, regardless of the value of "d."

Integer data (no decimal point in the input field) may also be read by E specification; in this case the "d" instruction serves to define the size of the resulting value. For example,

bbbbbb1234

would be interpreted by E10.2 as 12.34, but by E10.1 as 123.4.

Consistency between List and Specification Modes

In both input and output FORMAT statements, F and E specifications must be matched only with real variables in the input/output statement lists, and I specifications are valid only for integer variables. Execution error results from any mismatch. For example,

```
      WRITE (3,25) KING, ABLE, BAKER
   25 FORMAT (I10,F12.4)
```

fails in execution, because reuse of the FORMAT from the left parenthesis for the "extra" list variable (BAKER) calls for output of a real variable by way of an integer notation.

Consistency between Specifications and Input Data Modes

Our discussion of input FORMAT has indicated that the presence or absence of a decimal point in the input record field does not irrevocably define the data item as real or integer. A data item keypunched without decimal point may be read into a real location by an F or E specification (which supplies the decimal point location) or into an integer location by I specification. Thus

bbbbbb1234

may be interpreted as:

	12.34	(F10.2 or E10.2)
or	1234.0	(F10.0 or E10.0)
or	1234	(I10)
or	123	(I9)
or	12	(I8)
or	1	(I7)
or	0	(I6, I5, etc.)

Similarly, values appearing *with* decimal points in input data fields may be interpreted as real by way of F or E specifications or as integer by way of I specification. Thus

$$\text{bbbbb12.34}$$

may be read as:

	12.34	(Fw.d or Ew.d)
or	12	(I10, I9, I8, I7)
or	1	(I6)
or	0	(I5, I4, etc.)

This flexibility is reflected in many manufacturers' FORTRAN manuals by the use of the term *conversion* instead of "specification" or "notation": E conversion, F conversion, and so on.

Rounding Numbers for Output

If the stored value X = 1234.5678 is printed in

$$(Fw.2)$$

the value is truncated without rounding in most systems,[3] producing

$$1234.56$$

Furthermore, in binary computers a value such as 0.3 may be stored as 0.29999... and appear in output (Fw.2) as

$$0.29$$

---

[3] Some FORTRAN compilers, however, incorporate a rounding routine comparable to the programmer-supplied one described in this section. Check for its presence before attempting to use the suggested rounding arrangement.

Thus the programmer frequently has use for a simple technique that will produce properly rounded output.

Stored values may be corrected in advance of output by the addition of a rounding constant:

$$X = X + .005$$

Any X value that has a digit "5" or more in the *third* decimal location will thus be rounded upward, while no change would be produced in output for values containing lesser digits in the third location.

This rounding constant should obviously have a number of zeros equal to the "d" specification in FORMAT. Thus for Fw.4 the rounding constant is .00005, for Fw.0 it is .5, and so on.

Two kinds of error in using the technique should be avoided. First, values so adjusted should not be used subsequently for *computation* within the program, since they are no longer accurate in the unprinted decimal locations.

Second, simple addition will produce wrong-direction alteration for values in storage that are *negative*. This problem might be handled with an IF statement,

```
        -------------
        IF (X) 11,10,10
10      X = X + .005
        GO TO 12
11      X = X - .005
12      WRITE (3,108) X
108     FORMAT (F8.2)
        -------------
```

Another alternative that works, however, is

```
        -----------------
        X = X + .005 * (X/ABS(X))
        WRITE (3,108) X
        -----------------
```

Blank Columns (X), Output

The general form for transfer of blank characters is

$$nX$$

In this case, "n" cannot be omitted; an integer constant preceding "X" must be used to indicate the number of blanks. Thus

$$10X$$

creates ten blank output columns.

It is usually poor practice, in output FORMAT, to use the "X" instruction in front of F, E, or I notation specifications, since the generation of blanks preceding numeric output can be accomplished by providing extra room in the "w" portion of the specification. For example,

$$10XF5.1$$

should be written

$$F15.1$$

The second alternative is preferable because output values with large predecimal content, which may lead to execution errors (insufficient "w" size) when the first method is used, may fit within the second FORMAT's larger field.

We shall see some output use for the "X" instruction when we discuss transfer of alphameric characters.

Blank Columns (X), Input

The meaning of

$$10X$$

in an *input* FORMAT statement is "skip ten characters (columns) of the input record." The important function of such an instruction is the omission of material (alphabetic or numeric) that appears on input records but is not required as data for the program and therefore is not described by a variable name in the input statement list. For example, a card containing a product name (columns 1 to 15), a unit *price* (columns 16 to 25), a transactions figure (columns 26 to 35), and an inventory *quantity* (columns 36 to 45) may be read for just the price and quantity by

```
          READ (2,17) PRICE, QUANT
17     FORMAT (15XF10.2,10XF10.0)
```

Since the record portions that are to be eliminated are not blank, this *cannot* be accomplished by

```
17     FORMAT (25F10.2,20F10.0)
```

New Record (/), Output

Production of output on a set of three typed lines, printed lines, or punched cards is accomplished by the following statements:

```
        WRITE (M,18) K,A,B
18      FORMAT (I10/F15.4/F15.4)
```

Output of K is followed by shift to a new record (a new line at typewriter or printer or a new punched card). The second record (line) contains the A value and is followed by a third record containing B. Thus the output appearance is

```
        254
        13.1268
        11.2145
```

The effect on tape output is the placement of "end-of-record" marks following each output value. When the tape is used as input to a printing device, the final effect is thus the same as that shown above.

New Record (/), Input

A slash in FORMAT referenced by an input statement calls for a shift to the next input record. For example, the following statements read information from *four* successive punched cards:

```
        ------------------
        READ (2,19) L, M, A, FOX
19      FORMAT (2I5/F10.4//F5.0)
        ------------------
```

We have observed earlier that the execution of the READ statement itself causes selection of a new record. That is, the transfer of L and M is preceded by selection of a new card; L and M cannot be read from a card from which input data have been transferred earlier. Thus an input FORMAT statement that *begins* with a slash arranges the *skipping* of one record (card).

When L and M have been transferred, A is read from the *next* card; then a record is *skipped*, as the result of two successive slashes. The FOX value is then read from the fourth card. It is evident that k slashes arrange the skipping of (k − 1) complete records.

The use of the slash with reference to tape input has the same effect, the record-selection process being guided by the "end-of-record" marks mentioned earlier.

Mismatched Input Lists and Records

Length differences between the input *list* and the input *record* should be reconciled by the FORMAT statement. The "X" and "/" specifications are convenient for this purpose.

1. If the number of variables in the input list is less than the number of data items in each input record, "nX" may be used to bypass unwanted data items (as in our price-quantity example above).

2. If the input list contains *more* variables than there are data items on each record, the programmer must be sure to use "/" to indicate the necessary record shift. For example, with two data items per card,

```
      ┌ DO 13 K = 1, N
      │ READ (2,20) A, B, C, D
      │ ──────────────
      │ ──────────────
 13   └ ──────────────
 20     FORMAT (4F10.2)
```

will cause grave error. Two *blank* fields (to the right of actual data items) on each card will be stored as C = 0.00 and D = 0.00, at each execution of the READ statement. The situation can be cleared up by

20   FORMAT (2F10.2/2F10.2)

We have also noted earlier that this particular problem has another solution,

20   FORMAT (2F10.2)

which works because reuse of the FORMAT initiates selection of a new record. The latter solution is not available if the original statement says

20   FORMAT (2F10.2,2F5.0)

Transfer of Alphameric Characters

The FORMAT specifications we have discussed permit the transfer of *numeric* data only. Two major methods are available for the transfer of alphameric strings, which may include any combination of alphabetic, numeric, and special characters; these are "H" and "A" specifications.

Hollerith [4] (H) Strings and Literals, Output

The meaning of

$$nH$$

in FORMAT is "reproduce verbatim the following n characters." The "n" must be supplied as an integer constant, even for the value "1." This arranges the transfer of characters from within the FORMAT statement to the output medium.

The programmer may thus assign appropriate "labels" to describe numeric output. For example, the following segment arranges for a table caption and then produces the table itself in a single loop:

```
          WRITE (3,21)
     21   FORMAT (5X,21HNUMBER      SQUARE ROOT)
         ┌DO 30 K = 1,1000
         │X = K
         │X = X/10.0
         │S = SQRT(X) + .005
     30   └WRITE (3,50) X, S
     50   FORMAT (F10.1,F13.2)
```

(Note the use of the rounding constant.) The count represented by "n" must be exact and must include blank columns, since these are treated as characters that will be reproduced. Note that the "nX" instruction may be useful, in arranging blanks outside the Hollerith string. Furthermore, it may also be used to break the string into parts; statement 21 could be written by using "X" and "H" alternately:

```
     21   FORMAT (5X6HNUMBER4X11HSQUARE ROOT)
```

Some compilers (see Table 11) also permit the alphameric string to be enclosed by apostrophes (serving as quotation marks), in which case the nH

---

[4] Named for Herman Hollerith, the inventor of punch-card equipment.

TABLE 11

Transfer of Alphameric Characters

	Literal Transfer		A Format Maximum Field Width			No A Format
	Yes	No	Real	Integer	Either	
1[a]		✓				✓
2		✓			8	
3		✓	Depends on Control cards			
4		✓			6	
5	✓ "..."				6	
6	✓ '...'				4	
7		✓	Not allowed	2		
8		✓	6	4		
9		✓			8	
10		✓			2	
11		✓	8	4		
12		✓	8	4		
13	✓ *...*				8	
14		✓			10	
15	✓ *...*				10	
16		✓			4[b]	
17		✓	Not stated			
18		✓				✓
19		✓				✓
20	✓ "..."					✓
21		✓	5	Not allowed		
22	✓ '...'		5–10[c]	5		
23		✓	Not stated			
24		✓	Not stated			
25		✓				✓
26		✓	8	4		
27		✓	8	4		

[a] Compiler number.

[b] Extended by special rules.

[c] Second number applicable to double precision variables.

TABLE 11 (*continued*)

| | Literal Transfer | | A Format | | | No A |
| | Yes | No | Maximum Field Width | | | Format |
			Real	Integer	Either	
28		√				√
29	√ '...'		Not stated			
30		√			6	
31		√	6	3		
32		√			3	
33		√	8	4		
34		√			6	
35	√ $...$				63	
36	"..."^{d}		6	3		
37		√	Depends on control cards			
38		√	8	Not stated		
39		√	8–12^c	4		
40	√ '...'		4–8^c	4		
41	√ '...'					√
42	√ '...'		4–8^c	4		
43	√ '...'		Not stated			
44	√ '...'		4–6^c	2		
45		√	By control card	Not allowed		
46		√	Depends on control cards			
47		√	By control card	Not allowed		
48		√				√
49	√ '...'		4–6^c	2		
50		√	Depends on control cards			
51		√			6	
52		√			6	
53		√			5	
54		√				√
55		√			6	
56		√			8	
57		√	Not stated			

^{d} After PRINT, in output statement.

TABLE 11 (*continued*)

	Literal Transfer		A Format — Maximum Field Width			No A
	Yes	No	Real	Integer	Either	Format
58		√	Not stated			
59	√ $...$		10	8		
60		√	10–16^c	8	[Complex: 20]	
61		√			6^e	
62	[...]^d					√
63		√			6	
64	√ '...'		Not stated			
65		√			10	
66		√			10	
67		√	8	4		
68	√ '...' $...$		Not stated			
69	√ '...' $...$		Not stated			
70	√ '...'		Not stated			
71		√			2	
72		√			4	
73		√	6–9^c	3		
74	√ $...$		10	5		
75		√	10–16^c	3		
76		√			6	
77	√ '...'				6	
78		√	8	4		
79		√	No ruling			

^{e} 8 is installation option.

instruction is not necessary and the verbatim reproduction meaning is the same:

21   FORMAT ('   NUMBER   SQUARE ROOT')

This is known as *literal transfer*.

FORMAT statements may contain "labeling" information in combination with notation specifications for variables appearing in the output list. Thus we can produce as output

$$\text{MEAN} = \quad 15.2$$
$$\text{ST. DEV.} = \quad 1.6$$

by writing,

```
        WRITE (3,104) XMEAN, STDEV
104     FORMAT (11H     MEAN =F9.1/15H     ST. DEV. =F5.1)
```

Another useful technique, particularly for programs that are to be used as part of a program library, is the production of messages for the operator at execution time:

```
        WRITE (1,150)
        PAUSE
150     FORMAT ('PARAMETER N MUST PRECEDE DATA')
```

The PAUSE statement gives the operator the opportunity to check the data deck, after the reminder has been delivered.

Hollerith Strings, Input

The transfer of alphameric characters from an input medium *into a FORMAT statement* is also accomplished by nH or literals. The italics emphasize an important difference between this possibility and the "A" specification, discussed below. The only purpose of transferring alphameric information into a FORMAT statement is the subsequent reproduction of the entire unaltered string, in output. No manipulation of any kind is possible. Thus the following statements read in, and subsequently reproduce, a three-letter abbreviation for common stocks, which appears in columns 8, 9, and 10 of the card deck:

```
        ------------
       ┌DO 5 I = 1,N
       │READ (2,108) OPEN, CLOSE, VOL
       │------------------------
       │
       │------------------------
  5    └WRITE (3,108) GAIN, RATIO, FUND
108     FORMAT (7X3H     3F10.3)
        ------------------------
```

In this example, three columns in the FORMAT statement have been left blank, to be filled during execution. Any characters appearing in these FORMAT columns are replaced at each READ execution; therefore statement 108 could also have been written with

$$3H***$$
or   3HABC

and so on, so long as the correct count is preserved. An alternative for compilers permitting *literals* is

108   FORMAT (7X'***'3F10.3)

The Hollerith Constant

Some compilers permit the appearance of nH in two types of statement besides FORMAT. The CALL statement is discussed in Chapter 9 and the DATA statement in Chapter 11. The availability of the "Hollerith constant" for use in such statements is indexed in Table 25 (Chapter 11).

"A" Specifications

The "A" specification transfers alphameric characters between input/output media and *labeled storage*. The word "labeled" signifies that the storage location is referenced by one or more variable names. The general form is

$$nAw$$

in which "w" as usual represents the width of the data field; and "n" is optionally used for repeating specifications.

The instruction is analagous to

$$nIw$$

rather than to

$$nH$$

since the specification describes a field that is *mentioned as a variable in an input or output list*. If, for example, the common stock abbreviations in our last example were to be read in "A" FORMAT, the input and output statements must mention an additional variable, in the appropriate position:

```
--------------------
READ (2,1080) TITLE, OPEN, CLOSE, VOL
--------------------
WRITE (3,1080) TITLE, GAIN, RATIO, FUND
1080    FORMAT (7XA3,3F10.3)
--------------------
```

This usage, since it duplicates the performance of nH, does not suggest the real value of the "A" specification. Because the alphameric characters are actually stored in locations referenced by variable names, considerable manipulation is possible. Some of the manipulation techniques are discussed in Chapters 6, 10, 12, and 13. Some simpler possibilities include:

1. Input and output accomplished by separate FORMAT statements:

```
READ (2,110) NAME, AGE, GRADE
110    FORMAT (A6,2F10.0)
--------------------
WRITE (3,111) ANSWER, NAME
111    FORMAT (E15.7,10X,A6)
--------------------
```

2. Alteration of the string, between input and output:

```
READ (2,112) STATE
112    FORMAT (A10)
--------------------
WRITE (3,113) STATE
113    FORMAT (A3,1H.)
--------------------
```

3. Comparison of alphameric strings:

```
READ (2,130) NAME1, NAME2
130    FORMAT (2A5)
IF (NAME1 — NAME2)3,4,3
--------------------
```

The maximum permissible width of the "A" field varies from compiler to compiler and in many systems depends on whether the variable name used is integer or real. Table 11 shows applicable rules for various FORTRAN versions. When the maximum w is exceeded in input FORMAT, only the *rightmost* w characters in the input field will be transmitted. Note, however, that output resulting from "A" specification is usually *left*-justified, and output FORMAT that specifies a string shorter than that stored reproduces the *leftmost* characters from storage.

The limitation on size of w does not prevent the handling of longer strings, since variable titles may be combined. For example,

```
----------------------
        READ (2,150) PART1, PART2, PART3
150     FORMAT (3A10)
----------------------
        WRITE (3,151) XMEAN, PART1, PART2, PART3
151     FORMAT (F10.2, 3A10)
```

Printer Carriage Control

The on-line printer that most systems provide is frequently equipped with a vertical-movement control system that depends on instructions from the programmer. Such instructions are represented by the *first output character* that *would* be produced on an output record, as arranged by a given set of output and FORMAT statements. We say *"would"* because a character used for carriage control is then discarded, not printed. It would be printed *if* it were not being used for carriage control.

The most common arrangement (for exceptions, see Table 12) is:

First Output Character	Preprinting Carriage Movement
blank	single vertical space
0	double vertical space
1	space to new paper sheet
+	no vertical spacing
all others	interpreted as blank (single vertical space)

How have we controlled the printer carriage in our standard FORMAT statement

```
100     FORMAT (5F15.5)?
```

Our statement produces a single vertical space preceding printing (at each WRITE execution), because the extra room in "w" causes the printing of blank characters at the left of numeric output, including the critical first output character. A careful count would show, however, that the first blank is then lost,

TABLE 12

Printer Carriage Control

	Blank = Single Space	0 = Double Space	1 = Sheet Eject	+ = Suppress Space	1–9 = Skip to Channels 1–9	Other	None
1[a]							✓
2							✓
3	✓	✓		✓	✓		
4	✓	✓	✓			(Carriage movement *after* printing)	
5	✓	✓		✓	✓	(Carriage movement *after* printing)	
6							✓
7							✓
8	✓	✓	✓				
9	✓	✓	✓	✓		(Blank and + *after* printing)	
10	✓	✓	✓	✓			
11						20-character system; see Manufacturers' Manual, p. 9–26	
12							✓
13	✓	✓	✓				
14	✓	✓	✓	✓			
15	✓	✓	✓	✓			
16	✓	✓	✓	✓			
17						Statements: skip space	
18							✓
19							✓
20							✓
21	✓	✓	✓	✓			
22	✓	✓	✓	✓		7 additional characters; see Manufacturers' Manual, p. 31	
23	✓	✓	✓	✓			
24	✓	✓	✓	✓			
25							✓
26	✓	✓	✓	✓			
27	✓	✓	✓	✓	2–8 only		
28							✓
29	✓	✓	✓	✓			
30							✓
31	✓	✓	✓				
32	✓	✓	✓				
33						0 = skip/print/space 1 = eject/print/space	All others = print/space
34	✓	✓	✓	✓			
35							✓
36						In O/P statement, ↑ = new line	
37							✓
38	✓	✓	✓	✓			
39	✓	✓	✓			3 = suppress space	

[a] Compiler number.

TABLE 12 (*continued*)

	Blank = Single Space	0 = Double Space	1 = Sheet Eject	+ = Suppress Space	1–9 = Skip to Channels 1–9	Other	None
40	✓	✓	✓	✓			
41	✓	✓	✓	✓			
42	✓	✓	✓	✓			
43	✓	✓	✓	✓			
44	✓	✓	✓	✓			
45	✓	✓			✓		
46							✓
47	✓	✓			✓		
48	✓	✓			✓		
49	✓	✓	✓	✓			
50	✓				✓	K = double space L = triple space O, #, @ = channels 10, 11, 12.	b
51	✓	✓	✓				
52	✓	✓	✓				
53	✓	✓		✓	✓	J–L = short skip to channels 1–9	
54	✓	✓			✓		
55	✓	✓	✓				
56	✓	✓	✓	✓	2–7 only		
57	✓	✓	✓	✓			
58	✓	✓	✓	✓			
59							✓
60	✓	✓	✓	✓			
61	✓	✓	✓	✓			
62							✓
63	✓	✓	✓	✓			
64	✓	✓	✓	✓			
65	✓	✓	✓	✓		2 = vertical tab (tape loop)	
66	✓	✓	✓	✓		2 = vertical tab (tape loop)	
67							✓
68	✓	✓	✓	✓			
69	✓	✓	✓	✓			
70		✓	✓				
71	✓	✓	✓	✓			
72	✓	✓	✓	✓			
73	✓	✓	✓	✓			
74	✓	✓	✓	✓			
75	✓	✓	✓	✓			
76							✓
77	✓	✓	✓	✓			
78							✓
79	✓	✓	✓	✓			

b Also provides a set of after-printing characters; see Manufacturers' System Monitor Manual, p. 33.

so that the first value printed on any line occupies only 14 columns, not 15. The identical output could be produced by

1000   FORMAT (1H F14.5,4F15.5)

Alternatively, exactly 15 columns for each value would be obtained by

	1001	FORMAT (1H 5F15.5)
or by	1002	FORMAT (' '5F15.5)
or by	1003	FORMAT (1X,5F15.5)
or by	1004	FORMAT (9H NEW LINE5F15.5)
or by	1005	FORMAT (' NEW LINE'5F15.5)

These FORMAT statements all have in common the scheduling of a blank character for the first output column. Thus the *single space*, called for by a blank first output character, may actually be arranged in a number of ways: extra "w" room in F, I, or E specifications, H or literal specifications employed solely for the purpose, X instructions, and H or literal specifications beginning with a blank character and continuing for other purposes.

The "w" method is dangerous, however, since overly large output values (requiring 15 output columns) may create the single space (since characters other than those officially listed are interpreted as blanks), but at the cost of losing the first output digit, which will not be printed after use for carriage control.

The use of the "1H" specification for carriage control is most common in practice, since it does not alter subsequent specification counts and it can be employed for control characters *other than the blank*. For example,

10   FORMAT (1H + F10.1/1H0F20.1)

This arranges that the first value be printed on a line already used for output. Note that the instruction (1H0) for a vertical double space must be preceded by the slash, indicating commencement of a new record (print line). Conversely, the slash, when used in conjunction with the on-line printer, should be followed by a carriage control arrangement, since each new record is expected to begin with such an instruction.

It is interesting, though perhaps not very useful, to note that the "A" specification might be used to provide carriage control

----

WRITE (3,500) NOSPAC, A, B, C
500   FORMAT (A1,3F10.2)

This presupposes that NOSPAC has been read in "A" FORMAT earlier as "+."[5]

Planning Output FORMAT

We have mentioned earlier that execution errors may result from inadequate "w" size in FORMAT specifications. Even when mistakes in FORMAT do not provoke compiler or computer objections, they are annoying because sloppy-looking output resulting from minor errors requires recompiling of the entire program, after corrections have been made.

The best method of error avoidance is *planning of output with a sketch made on coding paper*. This permits direct translation into suitable specifications and is particularly useful for proper alignment of alphameric and numeric output. When the approximate size of output numbers is known beforehand, the sketch may be designed accordingly, with precision. When the ultimate size is in doubt, provision of extra space in "w," or use of exponential notation, may be appropriately arranged in the sketch. The use of coding paper for the purpose facilitates the exact column counts that are necessary for translation to FORMAT specifications. (However, output for 120-column printers should make use of 120-column paper, provided by some manufacturers as "printer layout paper").

As an example, let us arrange for the production of precisely the output shown in Fig. 14. The following program segment produces it:

```
       ----------------
       WRITE (3,10)
      ⌈DO 1 K = 1,N
      │READ (2,11) Q, P
      │V = Q * P
    1  ⌊WRITE (3,12) K, Q, P, V
   10   FORMAT (1H1,11X,3HN0.5X8HQUANTITY4X5HPRICE 7X5HVALUE/1H )
   12   FORMAT (I14,F12.0,F11.2,F14.2)

       ----------------
```

---

[5] Two other methods (besides reading as input) of defining an alphameric string in storage will be discussed later: the DATA statement in Chapter 10 and integer equivalence in Chapter 12.

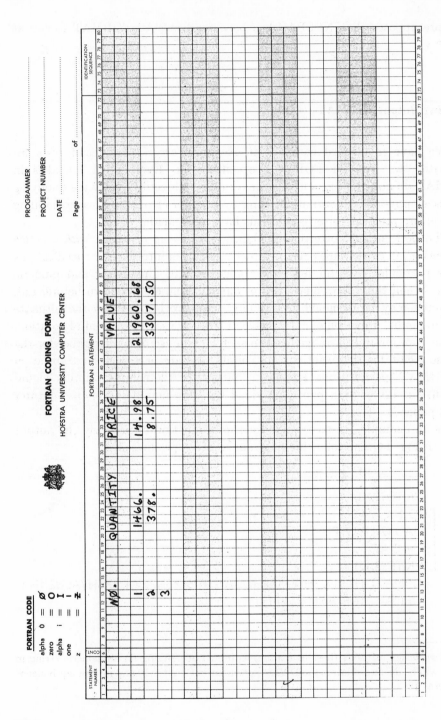

FIG. 14 Use of FORTRAN coding form for output planning.

Planning Input FORMAT

Input FORMAT is frequently dictated by the form of existing input records. For design of input FORMAT statements, data cards already keypunched thus serve the precise purpose described above for the coding-paper sketch of output form. That is, FORMAT specifications may be derived by direct copying from the card design.

For the special case of *alphameric* content on input records, our previous discussion provides the programmer with three alternatives:

1. nX "ignores" the alphameric fields.
2. nH reproduces the alphameric fields within the FORMAT statement.
3. nAw (used with variable name in the input list) reproduces the alphameric fields in storage locations referenced by variable names.

When the programmer does have the responsibility for design and organization of input data records, a guiding principle is that *uniformity* of data placement tends to keep the FORMAT statements few and short. Obviously, all cards in a data *deck* should follow the same field organization, so that a single FORMAT statement serves to describe them all. Furthermore, the use of standard field widths permits the use of a single repeated specification within that FORMAT statement. Thus a 100-card data deck, each card containing eight values, may be handled as simply as

```
     DO 15 L = 1, 100
     READ (2,300) A, B, C, D, E, F, G, H

     ---------------------

     ---------------------
15   ---------------------
300  FORMAT (8F10.4)

     ---------------------
```

We should observe, however, that some simplification of the input design problem must await the introduction of other FORTRAN techniques. For example, 100 values of a single variable would require 100 separate data cards, if reading and summation are done in this style:

```
     DO 111 M = 1, 100
     READ (2,120) X
111  SUM = SUM + X

     -----------------
```

We have explained earlier that repeated specifications in FORMAT statement 120 would have no effect, since only the first would be used at each READ execution.

This awkward size of the data deck cannot be reduced unless all values of X can be read in sequence, before summation is attempted. This implies that the 100 values must all be simultaneously in storage, which requires the *subscripted variable* (Chapter 7).

For Review	Examples
field	
field width	"w"
decimal portion of field	"d"
record	
numeric field	
alphameric field	
numeric specifications	
F notation	F10.2
I notation	I5
E notation	E16.7
repeated specification	3F10.2
repeated group of specifications	4(I5,E16.7)
right-justification	
conversion	
rounding constant	S = S + .005
positional specifications	
blank columns	10X
new record	/
alphameric specifications	
Hollerith string	6HMEAN =
literal transfer	'MEAN ='
A specification	3A5
carriage control characters	
single space	1Hb
double space	1H0
sheet eject	1H1
suppress space	1H+

EXERCISES

50. Keypunching errors frequently may be detected by checking to confirm that all data items are within a known allowable range. For example, IQ scores may range only from 0 to 300. Write a program that will

  (a) read a parameter indicating the number of data cards that follow (card #1; right-justified in columns 1–5);

(*b*) read low and high limits (real) for the data item to be checked (also on card #1, keypunched with decimal points, in columns 11–20 and 21–30);

(*c*) check through the deck for out-of-range items and print a suitable error message when any are encountered (message to include a sequence number for the errant item).

To test your program, keypunch the parameter card, using

$$15 \qquad -20. \qquad 80.$$

following FORMAT described in (*a*) and (*b*). Run on the entire data deck.

51. Write a program to read the *third* data item on each card and print out the (integer) position number (1–20) of each *negative* value. Output should read

ITEM NO.   IS NEGATIVE

ITEM NO.   IS NEGATIVE

etc.

52. Write a program that will read only the *fifth* data item, from only the *odd-numbered* data cards (1st, 3rd, . . ., 19th) and compute and print their arithmetic mean. The full data deck must be read. Let the output read precisely

MEAN   EXPONENTIAL FORM

xxx.xx   x.xxxxxxxE+xx

53. Since data cards out of sequence are a threat to any computer analysis, a useful program is one that simply checks a data deck to verify order. Write a program that will check integer sequence numbers keypunched in columns 73–80 (right-justified). When a card out of sequence is encountered, print the message

CARD OUT OF SEQUENCE FOLLOWING NUMBER—

and continue the testing process through the rest of the deck. (Make certain that a single card out of sequence does not generate more than one message.) The message should state the last card number that was in *correct* order. Do *not* assume that the sequence numbers must begin with "1"; but do assume that they increase by "1." The program should terminate when a *blank* card is encountered. Test your program on a six-card data deck sequenced 149, 150, 151, 159, 152, 153.

54. For any two variables for which quantitative observations are available, *correlation analysis* produces a *regression equation* describing the form of the function relating them, a *standard error of estimate* that summarizes dispersion of observations from the computed function, and a *coefficient of correlation* that evaluates the closeness of the relationship. Write a program that will compute these measures for n values of X and Y. Compute as follows:

(*a*) Regression coefficients:

$$b = \frac{n \sum XY - \sum X \sum Y}{n \sum X^2 - (\sum X)^2}$$

$$a = \overline{Y} - b\overline{X}$$

(b) Standard error of estimate:

$$S_{YX} = \sqrt{\frac{\sum Y^2 - a \sum Y - b \sum XY}{n}}$$

(c) Coefficient of correlation:

$$r = \sqrt{1 - \frac{S_{YX}^2}{\dfrac{\sum Y^2}{n} - \overline{Y}^2}}$$

Test your program on 20 observations. Each data card contains X in columns 1–15, and Y in columns 16–30.

55. Write a program to produce a table of X, $\log_e X$, and $\sqrt{X}$, with suitable caption labels, for X = 1.0, 1.1, 1.2, ..., 2.0. Round output values properly (unless your compiler does it automatically), printing *four* decimal places.

56. One of the problems in sports-car rallying (and automotive engineering tests) is to maintain driving speeds very precisely. To check whether a car is early or late, a "TSD Table" (time-speed-distance) is often used. The table shows, for a given speed, the time in minutes and seconds to travel a variety of distances. Write a program to compute such a table, for speeds from 45 to 65 mph (in steps of 1 mph). Show the elapsed time at each speed for distances 1.0, 2.5, and 5.0 miles. Arrange the table with suitable row and columns headings. Strive for typographical clarity so that it could be used easily by someone other than yourself.

57. Write a program that will copy *itself* on a printer, verbatim. That is, after the program is compiled, the source program itself will be reentered as data.

58. Write a program that reads the 20-card data deck, produces as output 20 arithmetic means (one per card; output to *two* decimal places, properly rounded), and also reproduces to the *left* of each mean the alphabetic information in columns 76–80.

59. A card deck contains customer names, keypunched as follows:

> columns 1–15   last name (left-justified)
> columns 16–30   first name (left-justified)

Write a program that will read the deck and reprint in the order: first initial—period—space—last name. For example,

JONES   JOHN

becomes

J. JONES

Make up and keypunch a four-card data deck to test the program.

60. Write a program that prints the *sum* of all the numeric items that appear on data cards containing a "B" in column 76 and/or an "L" in column 77. All decisions are to be made by the computer, not the programmer. The entire data deck must be read.

61. Write a program that reads the data deck and reprints only the *fourth* column, as a set of *integers* (no decimal point in output; postdecimal portions truncated). Also reprint the state names (columns 76–80) to the *right* of each output value. Use only one FORMAT statement in the program.

7 · SUBSCRIPTED VARIABLES

General Purpose and Method

The statement

$$\text{READ (IN,10) X}$$

has the effect, during compilation, of reserving a single storage location for the value "X." Yet we have seen that this statement during execution may actually handle many different values of X. Our frequent looping arrangement

```
   ┌DO 1 K = 1,N
   │READ (IN,10) X
1  └SUM = SUM + X
```

repeatedly replaces old values of X with new ones as the reading proceeds. After exit from the loop, the only value of X *in storage* is the last one read—the nth value.

The purpose of *subscripting* is the simultaneous retention in storage of multiple values of any variable. The method is precisely analogous to mathematical notation;

$$X_1, X_2, X_3, X_4, \ldots, X_n$$

becomes in FORTRAN

$$\text{X(1), X(2), X(3), X(4), \ldots, X(N)}$$

The entire set of values thus designated is frequently referred to as an *array*; individual values are *array elements*.

As an example of the technique, let us write a program to compute the *standard deviation* of 100 values, by the definitional method (square root of the average squared deviation from the arithmetic mean),

$$S_X = \sqrt{\frac{\sum (X - \bar{X})^2}{n}}$$

Subscripting is necessary, since individual values of X must be available for computation of deviations from the arithmetic mean, *after* the latter has been produced.

```
C       STANDARD DEVIATION—100 ITEMS
        DIMENSION X(100)
        SUM = 0.
       ┌DO 1 K = 1, 100
       │READ (2,100) X(K)
1      └SUM = SUM + X(K)
        XM = SUM/100.
        SUM = 0.
       ┌DO 2 JOE = 1, 100
2      └SUM = SUM + (X(JOE) − XM)**2
        STDEV = SQRT(SUM/100.) + .00005
        WRITE (3,101) STDEV
100     FORMAT (F10.2)
101     FORMAT (1H 10HST. DEV. =,F14.4)
        CALL EXIT
        END
```

The programmer's intention to store multiple values of a variable must be expressed at the beginning of the source program, by use of a DIMENSION statement (a *nonexecutable specification* statement). If, however, a variable that is to be subscripted is also to be "typed" by an explicit specification statement (REAL or INTEGER), its dimensions should be declared in the type statement, which *precedes* any DIMENSION statements. Dimension information so appearing should not be repeated in DIMENSION. For example,

```
REAL ITEM(10)
INTEGER PROD(20), CLIMB(20)
DIMENSION FAULT(20)
```

The DIMENSION statement in the STANDARD DEVIATION program has the effect during compilation of setting aside 100 floating-point (real) locations in storage and referencing these as $X_1, X_2, X_3, X_4, \ldots, X_{100}$. A statement declaring the dimensionality *must* appear prior to the first mention of a variable that is to be subscripted. Conversely, any variable declared to be an array (in a DIMENSION or type statement)[1] must be provided with a subscript each time it is mentioned in the source program.[2]

The parentheses of the DIMENSION statement must contain an integer *constant*. An integer variable is not acceptable, even when previously defined.[3] The reason for this requirement should be obvious: the reservation of storage locations for all variables is a *compilation* activity, and variables are not represented by actual values in storage until *execution* time. The statement

$$J = 100$$

is translated to machine language during compilation, and a storage location is reserved for J. But that storage location is still empty at the end of compilation; it is filled during execution. Therefore

DIMENSION X(J)

is not valid.

Permissible Subscript Forms

The subscript appears in parentheses immediately following the name of the variable being subscripted and is treated as a part of that name. The subscript must be in *integer mode*—either an integer constant, an integer variable, or one of a *limited* set of more complex integer expressions. In most FORTRAN compilers, the acceptable forms of integer expression are the following (v represents any integer variable; c and d represent any integer constants):

	General Form	Example
(1)	v	X(K)
(2)	c	X(36)
(3)	v + c	X(K + 2)
(4)	v − c	X(JOB − 5)
(5)	c * v	X(2*M)
(6)	c * v + d	X(2*M+1)
(7)	c * v − d	X(4*LUMP−3)

---

[1] In addition to REAL, INTEGER, and DIMENSION, another statement that may contain the dimension information, COMMON, is discussed in Chapter 9, and three other type specification statements that may also serve the purpose (DOUBLE PRECISION, COMPLEX, LOGICAL) are discussed in Chapter 10.

[2] An exception for input and output statements appears later in this chapter.

[3] An exception, for subprograms, is discussed in Chapter 9.

In types (3) through (7), the *order* of these expressions must be rigidly adhered to. That is, the following examples do *not* contain valid subscripts:

$$X(3 + K)$$
$$X(K*3)$$
$$X(6 + 3*K)$$

Although some compilers permit the appearance as subscript of *any* integer expression and others go further to include the use of subscripts in *real* mode, restriction to the seven forms shown assures intercomputer compatibility for your programs. Table 13 shows permissible subscript forms for various FORTRAN compilers.

TABLE 13

Permissible Subscript Forms

	V	C	V + C V − C	C * V	C * V + D C * V − D	Any Integer Expression	Any Arithmetic Expression	Not Stated
1[a]	√	√	√	√	√			
2	√	√	√	√	√			
3	√	√	√	√	√			
4	√	√	√	√	√	√	√	
5	√	√	√	√	√	√	√	
6	√	√	√	√	√	√		
7	√	√	√	√	√			
8	√	√	√	√	√			
9	√	√	√	√	√	√[b]	√[b]	
10	√	√	√	√	√			
11	√	√	√	√	√			
12	√	√	√	√	√			
13	√	√	√	√	√	√[b]	√[b]	
14	√	√	√	√	√			
15	√	√	√	√	√	√[b]	√[b]	
16								√
17	√	√	√	√	√	√	√	
18	√	√	√	√	√			

[a] Compiler number.
[b] Except in I/O statement; USAS only.

TABLE 13 (*continued*)

	V	C	V + C V − C	C ∗ V	C ∗ V + D C ∗ V − D	Any Integer Expression	Any Arithmetic Expression	Not Stated
19		√						
20	√	√	√	√	√	√		
21	√	√	√	√	√			
22	√	√	√	√	√	√		
23	√	√	√	√	√			
24	√	√	√	√	√			
25	√	√	√	√	√			
26	√	√	√	√	√	√		
27	√	√	√	√	√			
28	√	√	√	√	√			
29	√	√	√	√	√			
30	√	√	√	√	√			
31	√	√	√	√	√	√	√	
32	√	√	√	√	√			
33	√	√	√	√	√			
34	√	√	√	√	√			
35	√	√	√	√	√	√	√	
36	√	√	√	√	√	√	√	
37	√	√	√	√	√			
38	√	√	√	√	√			
39	√	√	√	√	√	√		
40	√	√	√	√	√			
41	√	√	√	√	√			
42	√	√	√	√	√	√	√ [except complex]	
43	√	√	√	√	√			
44	√	√	√	√	√			
45	√	√	√	√	√			
46	√	√	√	√	√			
47	√	√	√	√	√			
48	√	√	√					

TABLE 13 (*continued*)

	V	C	V + C V − C	C * V	C * V + D C * V − D	Any Integer Expression	Any Arithmetic Expression	Not Stated
49	√	√	√	√	√			
50	√	√	√	√	√			
51	√	√	√	√	√			
52	√	√	√	√	√			
53	√	√	√	√	√			
54	√	√	√	√	√			
55	√	√	√	√	√			
56	√	√	√	√	√	√		
57	√	√	√	√	√	√		
58	√	√	√	√	√	√		
59	√	√	√	√	√	√	√	
60	√	√	√	√	√	√	√	
61	√	√	√	√	√			
62	√	√	√	√	√	√		
63	√	√	√	√	√			
64	√	√	√	√	√			
65	√	√	√	√	√			
66	√	√	√	√	√			
67	√	√	√	√	√			
68	√	√	√	√	√	√	√	
69	√	√	√	√	√	√	√	
70	√	√	√	√	√			
71	√	√	√	√	√			
72	√	√	√	√	√			
73	√	√	√	√	√			
74	√	√	√	√	√			
75	√	√	√	√	√			
76	√	√	√	√	√	√		
77	√	√	√	√	√	√		
78	√	√	√	√	√			
79	√	√	√	√	√			

In the sample program (STANDARD DEVIATION), only the first form, the single integer variable, is used. The usefulness of the DO statement in conjunction with subscripted variables is evident. The DO *Index* serves as a convenient subscript, since (*a*) it is in the proper mode and (*b*) it "automatically" represents a changing series of values, in this case the values 1 through 100. The second execution of the READ statement does not cause erasure of the first X value in storage, simply because the first READ execution is in effect

$$\text{READ (2,100) X(1)}$$

and the second is executed as

$$\text{READ (2,100) X(2)}$$

Since the computer locates the array elements in storage by subscript *number*, the programmer is not committed, in later parts of the program, to repetition of the original integer variable used as subscript. Thus JOE appears as the second DO Index in the sample program, and also serves as subscript.

Both real and integer variables may be subscripted; in either case, the subscripts themselves must be in integer mode.[4] A single DIMENSION statement may mention any number of variables that are to be subscripted. For example, the following program produces three percentage distributions, an activity requiring subscripting because the original data items are required for computations based on the three sums; and the sums are fully formed only after all data have been read.

```
C       THREE COLUMNS, PERCENT DISTRIBUTIONS VERTICALLY
        DIMENSION REPUB(200), DEMO(200), CONS(200)
        SREP = 0
        SDEM = 0
        SCON = 0
        WRITE (2,99)
       ⌈DO 2 M = 1,200
        │READ (2,100) REPUB(M), DEMO(M), CONS(M)
        │IF (REPUB(M) − 9999.99)1,3,3
      1 │SREP = SREP + REPUB(M)
        │SDEM = SDEM + DEMO(M)
      2 ⌊SCON = SCON + CONS(M)
```

---

[4] In those systems that permit *real* expressions as subscripts, the final expression value is truncated to integer form.

```
3       K = M−1
       ┌DO 4 J = 1,K
       │P1 = REPUB(J)/SREP*100.+.005
       │P2 = DEMO(J)/SDEM*100.+.005
       │P3 = CONS(J)/SCON*100.+.005
4      └WRITE (2,100) P1, P2, P3
        CALL EXIT
99      FORMAT (4X3HREP7X3HDEM7X3HCON/)
100     FORMAT (3F10.2)
        END
```

Some techniques that we have discussed earlier are also visible in this program:

1. The output table is preceded by a row of column titles, arranged in FORMAT statement 99.

2. The first DO loop contains an IF statement, which tests for a sentinel card containing a dummy data item (9999.99). Thus the program is designed to perform on varying numbers of data items. However, the necessity of providing integer *constants* in the DIMENSION statement forces us to limit the program to some *maximum* (200) number of data cards. When the program is executed for a smaller data set, some of the storage reserved for the array will remain empty.

3. Rounding of output values is accomplished in the second DO loop, by a technique discussed in the last chapter.

An interesting problem that requires subscripting is the internal *ranking* of values (also called *sorting*)—that is, rearrangement to order them from low to high or high to low. There are literally hundreds of methods for accomplishing this. A basic technique, which is slower than many others in execution, but logically simple, involves a sequence of comparisons designed in accordance with the "COMBINATIONS" program segment at the end of Chapter 5. The sorting is accomplished by comparing

$$X_1 \text{ \& } X_2$$
$$X_1 \text{ \& } X_3$$
$$X_1 \text{ \& } X_4$$
$$- - - - - -$$
$$X_1 \text{ \& } X_n$$

Each such comparison is followed by *interchange* of the two storage positions, *if* the array element on the left is higher than the right-hand element. The first set of comparisons thus moves the lowest X value to the X(1) location. The next set of comparisons is performed as

$$X_2 \ \& \ X_3$$
$$X_2 \ \& \ X_4$$
$$X_2 \ \& \ X_5$$
$$\text{-----}$$
$$X_2 \ \& \ X_n$$

This process must be repeated (n − 1) times, ending with the comparison

$$X_{n-1} \ \& \ X_n$$

For n values (using a parameter card), the program appears as follows:

```
C     RANKING—METHOD 1
      INTEGER START
      DIMENSION X(500)
C     READ PARAMETER
      READ (2,10) N
C     READ X VALUES
      DO 1 I = 1, N
1     READ (2,11) X(I)
C     ARRANGE FOR (N−1) COMPARISON SETS
      LIM = N − 1
      DO 3 I = 1, LIM
C     ARRANGE STARTING POINT FOR EACH SET
      START = I + 1
C     BEGIN COMPARISON SET
      DO 3 J = START, N
      IF (X(I) − X(J)) 3, 3, 2
C     INTERCHANGE POSITIONS IN STORAGE
2     SAVE = X(I)
      X(I) = X(J)
      X(J) = SAVE
3     CONTINUE
C     OUTPUT AND EXIT
      DO 4 I = 1, N
4     WRITE (3,11) X(I)
      CALL EXIT
10    FORMAT (I4)
11    FORMAT (F12.2)
      END
```

Some features of this program should be reviewed:

1. FORMAT statement 10 specifies integer notation, since the parameter is being read (and used) in integer mode.

2. The third DO statement would not be legal, without the *explicit type specification* statement.

3. Two DO loops end on the same statement, a permissible arrangement that gives precedence to execution of the inner loop.

4. The CONTINUE statement is made necessary by the required branch to the bottom of the nest of loops, for data items already in "correct" order.

5. The technique for *interchanging* the locations of two values in storage should be studied. A simple two-statement arrangement would *not* work:

$$X(I) = X(J)$$
$$X(J) = X(I)$$

It would merely produce two values both equal to the original value of $X(J)$. "SAVE" is a location used to hold the value of $X(I)$ for use in the third statement that completes the interchange.

Input/Output with Subscripted Variables

The data for the last sample program ("RANKING") must be keypunched one item per card, and the output will appear as a single column of values. Several methods are available for reduction of the size of the data deck and for arrangement of multiple output on each line.

One such method makes use of the "adjusted" subscript—that is, a subscript containing simple arithmetic. For data keypunched five items per card,

```
       ──────────────────
     ┌DO 4 L = 1, 100, 5
  4  └READ (2,10) X(L), X(L+1), X(L+2), X(L+3), X(L+4)
 10     FORMAT (5F10.2)
       ──────────────────
```

Note the use of the DO loop increment (5). The second execution translates to

```
READ (2,10) X(6), X(7), X(8), X(9), X(10)
```

The same output list may be specified more conveniently, however, by using a statement form variously called *implied DO loop* or *indexed list*. The form is valid only for *input* or *output* statements; it consists of inclusion within such a statement of an Index (an integer variable, as in the DO statement) and starting value, limit, and increment (integer variables or constants) for the Index. For example,

$$\text{READ (2,10) (X(L), L = 1, 100)}$$

has exactly the same effect as the entire DO loop in the last sample segment, the FORMAT statement remaining the same. [Note, however, that the increment (5) is *not* required and would in fact cause error.] An important difference, however, is that the *indexed list* version calls for just *one* execution of the READ statement. Therefore the data may be in any number of fields per record; the FORMAT statement controls the choice of the next card (by specifying "5" in front of "F" in the example).

If the programmer actually wants some subscript values skipped, the increment may be useful. This may be illustrated by an output statement that punches only odd-subscripted array elements, producing seven values per output line:

$$\text{WRITE (2,12) (X(M), M = 1, N, 2)}$$
$$\text{12 \quad FORMAT (7F10.2)}$$

Another useful possibility is available when *all* elements of an array are to be transferred by an input or output statement. The word "all" as used here signifies *agreement in number with the constant in the DIMENSION statement*. It is then permissible to *omit* the subscript entirely, an omission that will be interpreted as specifying the *entire array* (in ascending subscript order). For example,

$$\text{DIMENSION X(350)}$$
$$\text{READ (2,13) X}$$
$$\text{13 \quad FORMAT (7F7.3)}$$

This segment will handle a 50-card data deck, executing as though the READ statement said

$$\text{READ (2, 13) (X(I), I = 1, 350)}$$

Remember that these two arrangements—the indexed list and subscript omission—are valid only in input and output statements. The convenience offered by these methods suggests that subscripting of a variable may be worthwhile even for instances in which each value need be used only once in the

program. That is, the data deck and/or the input and output statements may be
shortened by such practice. Compare the following segments:

(1)
```
        --------------------
       ┌ DO 1 K = 1, 800
       │ READ (2,14) X              Data deck: 800 cards
   1   └ SUM = SUM + X
   14    FORMAT (F8.2)
        --------------------
```

(2)
```
     --------------------
    ┌ DO 1 K = 1,100             Data deck: 100 cards
    │ READ (2,15) XA, XB, XC, XD, XE, XF, XG, XH
  1 └ SUM = SUM + XA + XB + XC + XD + XE + XF + XG + XH
  15   FORMAT (8F8.2)
     --------------------
```

(3)
```
     --------------------
      DIMENSION X(800)
      READ (2,16) X
    ┌ DO 1 K = 1,800             Data deck: 100 cards
  1 └ SUM = SUM + X(K)
  16   FORMAT (8F8.2)
```

Table 14 shows availability of the indexed list and subscript omission for arrays,
in input and output statements. (The table also deals with multiple subscripts,
discussed below.)

A situation in which the "A" FORMAT specification is useful in conjunction with subscripted variables occurs when a specific FORMAT statement is
to be used for repetitive output, changing only an alphameric portion. The use
of "H" or "literals" (' ') in this situation would necessitate a large number of
FORMAT *and* WRITE statements (since the FORMAT statement number
cannot be written as a variable):

```
        --------------------
        WRITE (3,100) POP, TEMP, ALT
  100   FORMAT (1H 'ALA.'3F15.0)
        --------------------
        WRITE (3,101) POP, TEMP, ALT
  101   FORMAT (1H 'ARIZ.'3F15.0)
        --------------------
        WRITE (3,102) POP, TEMP, ALT
  102   FORMAT (1H 'ARK.'3F15.0)
        --------------------
```

TABLE 14

Input/Output of Arrays—Maximum Array Dimensions

	Indexed List		Subscript Omission		Maximum Dimensions					
	Yes	No	Yes	No	2	3	7	Unlimited	Other	Not Stated
1[a]	✓		✓		✓					
2	✓		✓			✓				
3	✓		✓			✓				
4	✓		✓			✓				
5	✓		✓					✓		
6	✓		✓				✓			
7	✓		✓			✓				
8	✓		✓			✓				
9	✓		✓			✓				
10	✓		✓			✓				
11	✓		✓			✓				
12	✓		✓			✓				
13	✓		✓			✓				
14	✓		✓			✓				
15	✓		✓			✓				
16	✓		✓			✓				
17	✓		✓			✓				
18	✓		✓		✓					
19		✓		✓	✓					
20		✓		✓					1	
21	✓			✓		✓				
22	✓		✓					✓		
23	✓		✓			✓				
24	✓		✓				✓			
25		✓	✓		✓					
26	✓		✓			✓				
27	✓		✓			✓				
28	✓		✓		✓					
29	✓		✓				✓			
30	✓		✓			✓				

[a] Compiler number.

TABLE 14 (*continued*)

	Indexed List		Subscript Omission		Maximum Dimensions					
	Yes	No	Yes	No	2	3	7	Unlimited	Other	Not Stated
31	√		√						20	
32	√		√		√					
33	√		√			√				
34	√		√				√			
35	√		√					√		
36	√		√						15^b	
37	√			√	√					
38	√		√			√				
39	√		√					√		
40	√		√			√				
41	√		√			√				
42	√		√				√			
43	√		√				√			
44	√		√			√				
45	√		√		√					
46	√		√			√				
47	√		√			√				
48		√		√	√					
49	√		√			√				
50	√		√			√				
51	√		√			√				
52	√		√			√				
53	√		√			√				
54	√		√			√				
55	√		√				√			
56	√		√						32	
57	√		√					√		
58	√		√					√		
59	√		√							√
60	√		√							$√^c$

[b] Maximum of 8191 locations.

[c] Up to 3 shown in Manufacturers' Manual examples.

TABLE 14 (*continued*)

	Indexed List		Subscript Omission		Maximum Dimensions					
	Yes	No	Yes	No	2	3	7	Unlimited	Other	Not Stated
61	√		√			√				
62		√		√		√				
63	√		√				√			
64	√		√				√			
65	√		√			√				
66	√		√			√				
67	√		√			√				
68	√		√					√		
69	√		√					√		
70	√		√				√			
71	√		√			√				
72	√		√			√				
73	√		√			√				
74	√		√			√				
75	√		√			√				
76	√		√					√		
77	√		√					√		
78	√		√			√				
79	√		√			√				

The state abbreviations in this example may be read in "A" FORMAT (let us allow a maximum of five characters and keypunch them sixteen per card), and then incorporated in output by a single set of WRITE and FORMAT statements:

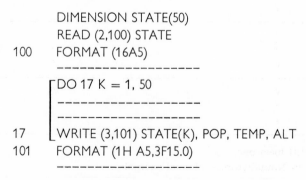

```
        DIMENSION STATE(50)
        READ (2,100) STATE
100     FORMAT (16A5)
        - - - - - - - - - - - - - - - - - -
       ┌DO 17 K = 1, 50
       │ - - - - - - - - - - - - - - - - -
       │ - - - - - - - - - - - - - - - - -
17     └WRITE (3,101) STATE(K), POP, TEMP, ALT
101     FORMAT (1H A5,3F15.0)
        - - - - - - - - - - - - - - - - - -
```

Double Dimension

It is possible in FORTRAN to assign *two* subscripts to a dimensioned variable. This arrangement must be mentioned in the DIMENSION statement (or the *type* statement used for declaring dimensionality)—and, conversely, each time a variable so treated appears in the program[5] it must be identified with two subscripts. The statement

$$\text{DIMENSION W(3,4)}$$

reserves storage for *twelve* values of W. They will be referenced as

$$X_{1,1}, \ X_{2,1}, \ X_{3,1}, \ X_{1,2}, \ X_{2,2}, \ X_{3,2}, \ X_{1,3}, \ \ldots, \ X_{3,4}$$

This is also the order (referred to below as *column* order) in which the computer assigns sequential storage for the two-dimensional array. Note that the *first* subscript varies *first*.

The reason for election of this method in preference to

$$\text{DIMENSION W(12)}$$

is the programmer's conceptual view of the data as a two-dimensional matrix in which identification of each value by two coordinates or characteristics is convenient. Some examples of problems generating such data may illustrate this point:

Economics: data representing m industries in n different years.
Mathematics: data representing m simultaneous equations, each containing n variables.
Business data processing: data representing m products, each subject to n transactions.
Statistics: data representing two categorical variables, one with m values and the other with n values.
Survey research: data representing m respondents, each answering n questions.
Engineering: data representing m materials, each having n characteristics.

The usual permissible forms of the subscript are usable in double dimension. Thus the following are all valid:

$$\text{W(L,ML)}$$
$$\text{W(3,2)}$$
$$\text{W(ITEM, K+6)}$$
$$\text{W(3*K+1, N-6)}$$

---

[5] With the exception of the input/output "subscript omission" arrangement.

The use of a double dimension arrangement is facilitated by the programmer's adherence to a fixed organizational reference method for the data. One such organization is the use of the first subscript to designate *rows* (horizontal) and the second to designate *columns* (vertical) of data. That is, the 3×4 array of W in our illustration is conceived as

$$
\begin{array}{cccc}
W_{1,1} & W_{1,2} & W_{1,3} & W_{1,4} \\
W_{2,1} & W_{2,2} & W_{2,3} & W_{2,4} \\
W_{3,1} & W_{3,2} & W_{3,3} & W_{3,4}
\end{array}
$$

It is also convenient to retain a fixed subscript (i) to indicate row number and another subscript (j) to indicate column number. Within this framework, the double DO loop (i.e., a two-deep "nest") may be used to travel through the data either *horizontally*

```
      ┌─DO 1 I = 1,3        (rows)       Order:
      │  DO 1 J = 1,4        (columns)    1,1  1,2  1,3  1,4
      │  ┌──────W(I,J)                       etc.
   1  └──└────────────
```

or *vertically*

```
      ┌─DO 2 J = 1,4        (columns)   Order:
      │  DO 2 I = 1,3        (rows)         1,1  etc.
      │  ┌──────W(I,J)                      2,1
   2  └──└───────────                       3,1
```

The change in direction is accomplished by simple reversal of the DO statements. As an example, the following segments both obtain the same sum:

```
         ─────────────────
         ACROSS = 0
      ┌─DO 1 I = 1,3
      │ ┌─DO 1 J = 1,4
   1  └─└─ACROSS = ACROSS + W(I,J)
         ─────────────────
         DOWN = 0
      ┌─DO 2 J = 1,4
      │ ┌─DO 2 I = 1,3
   2  └─└─DOWN = DOWN + W(I,J)
```

Indexed List and Subscript Omission for Double Dimension

While the double DO loop is convenient for computation, input/output activities may take advantage of the *indexed list* and *subscript omission* features. That is, we may substitute for:

```
        DIMENSION X(15,10)
       ┌DO 1 I = 1, 15
       │┌DO 1 J = 1, 10
    1  └└READ (2,10) X(I,J)
   10     FORMAT (10F8.4)
   -----------------------
```

This arrangement would require data keypunched one item per card. (Nine of the ten specifications in FORMAT statement 10 are simply ignored, at each execution of the READ statement.) The double-loop effect may be duplicated for more closely packed data (ten items per card, same FORMAT) by:

$$\text{READ (2,10) ((X(I,J), J = 1, 10), I = 1, 15)}$$

In this method, the Index mentioned first is the first to change (i.e., is treated as the *inner* implied DO loop Index). Therefore, the statement shown treats the variable in what we have defined as "horizontal" (or "row") order. Input design and FORMAT statement are now correctly matched.

To write the 15 × 10 matrix as a 10 × 15 *transpose*,[6] the index positions are reversed:

```
        WRITE (3,12) ((X(I,J), I = 1, 15), J = 1, 10)
   12     FORMAT (1H 15F8.4)
```

As in the case of the single-dimensioned variable, the *omission* of all subscripts from an *input* or *output* statement in which the variable is listed will have the effect of specifying the entire array, as dimensioned. The order, however, is by *columns* (the first subscript changing first, as stored internally). This is the order that we have defined as "vertical." That is, our last WRITE statement could be duplicated as

$$\text{WRITE (3,12) X}$$

---

[6] The *transpose* of

1	2	3	4
5	6	7	8
9	10	11	12

is

1	5	9
2	6	10
3	7	11
4	8	12

Single Loops for Double Dimension

A single DO loop may also be useful in input or output of double-dimensioned variables, particularly in conjunction with an indexed list that implies the other loop. For example, if each data card in our last set contains an initial field that is to be read as alphameric material,

```
        ┌DO 155 I = 1,15
    155  └READ (2,14) TITLE(I),(X(I,J),J=1,10)
    14      FORMAT (A6,10F7.3)
```

You should keep in mind the possibility of combining the best features of each of these methods, as convenience dictates. For example, a program to compute row and column sums for a specific 3 × 4 matrix (three rows, four columns) may be written as follows, for data punched on a single card in "vertical" order and output printed in "horizontal" order. The program utilizes subscript omission for input and for output of column sums, a single-loop arrangement with indexed list for other output, and the double-loop arrangement for summation.

```
    C      ROW AND COLUMN SUMS, 3 BY 4
           DIMENSION F(3,4), SR(3), SC(4)
           ┌DO 1 I = 1,3
    1      └SR(I) = 0
           ┌DO 2 J = 1,4
    2      └SC(J) = 0
           READ (2,10) F
          ┌─DO 3 I = 1,3
          │┌DO 3 J = 1,4
          ││SR(I) = SR(I) + F(I,J)
    3     └└SC(J) = SC(J) + F(I,J)
           ┌DO 4 I = 1,3
    4      └WRITE (3,11) (F(I,J),J=1,4), SR(I)
           WRITE (3,12) SC
    10     FORMAT (12F5.0)
    11     FORMAT (1H 4F5.0,F7.0)
    12     FORMAT (1H0,4F5.0)
           CALL EXIT
           END
```

If the program were to be *generalized* for an m × n matrix, we would have the following:

1. The DIMENSION statement would be altered to indicate a *maximum* number of rows and columns; for example,

$$\text{DIMENSION F(20,20), SR(20), SC(20)}$$

2. All limiting constants "3" could be replaced by "M" and all limiting constants "4" by "N."

3. The parameters M and N could be read from a card preceding the data:[7]

$$\text{READ (2,13) M, N}$$
$$13 \quad \text{FORMAT (2I3)}$$

4. The data-reading statement would require alteration, since the entire dimensioned array need not appear as data. A simple solution is

$$\text{READ (2,10) ((F(I,J),J=1,N),I=1,M)}$$

Triple Dimension

Many FORTRAN compilers permit the use of *three* subscripts to identify values of a variable (and some allow even more; see Table 14). By analogy to the double-dimension discussion, you should readily comprehend the possible arrangements:

$$\text{DIMENSION M(4,5,6)}$$

reserves storage for 120 values of M. The values might be read (one item punched per card) by way of a triple DO loop set:

```
      ┌─DO 1 I = 1,4
      │ ┌─DO 1 J = 1,5
      │ │ ┌DO 1 K = 1,6
   1  └─└─└READ (2,10) M(I,J,K)
  10      FORMAT (I2)
```

---

[7] Since reference to a subscript value higher than that appearing in DIMENSION causes serious execution error, additional checking statements are good practice; for example,

$$\text{IF (M − 20) 90, 90, 91}$$
$$90 \quad \text{IF (N − 20) 1, 1, 91}$$

in which statement 91 produces an error message and an execution halt.

The same work performed with an indexed list:

$$\text{READ (2,11) ((((M(I,J,K), K = 1,6), J=1,5), I=1,4)}$$
$$11 \quad \text{FORMAT (30I2)}$$

And, finally, the entire array might be read in via subscript omission:

$$\text{READ (2,12) M}$$
$$12 \quad \text{FORMAT (30I2)}$$

In the last instance, the effective order of treatment will be opposite to the prior indexed-list version; that is, it is equivalent to

$$\text{READ (2,11) (((M(I,J,K) I=1,4), J=1,5), K=1,6)}$$

Although it is not convenient to conceive of a triple-dimension array in simple terms of "rows" and "columns," there are many instances of three-dimensional data sets.

For example, employment data for ten industries, each with 32 occupation classifications, for each of four years, may be handled by

$$\text{DIMENSION E(10,32,4)}$$

This reserves storage for 1,280 E values, which are each identified by three subscripts. Thus

$$\text{E(4,11,3)}$$

represents the fourth industry, eleventh occupation, in the third year. If data are keypunched by industry,

	(1950)	(1955)	(1960)	(1965)
(occupation 1)	xxxxx	xxxxx	xxxxx	xxxxx
(occupation 2)	xxxxx	xxxxx	xxxxx	xxxxx
(occupation 32)	xxxxx	xxxxx	xxxxx	xxxxx

then the "year" subscript should change first, the occupation subscript second, and the industry subscript last, as the data are read in. This may be accomplished by

$$\text{READ (2,10)(((E(I,J,K),K=1,4),J=1,32),I=1,10)}$$
$$10 \quad \text{FORMAT (4F10.0)}$$

We may observe, however, that a rearrangement in the DIMENSION statement would permit the use of the subscript-omission method, without altering
our assignment of meaning to the subscripts:

```
DIMENSION E(4,32,10)
READ (2,10) E
```

Total employment for each year could be computed by use of a triple DO
loop:

```
      DIMENSION E(4,32,10), TOTAL(10,4)
      READ (2,10) E
    ┌─DO 1 K = 1, 10
    │┌─DO 1 I = 1, 4
    ││  TOTAL(K,I) = 0.
    ││┌─DO 1 J = 1, 32
1   └┴┴  TOTAL(K,I) = TOTAL(K,I) + E(I,J,K)
```

Output of the 40 totals might then be arranged as

	(1950)	(1955)	(1960)	(1965)
(Industry) 1				
(Industry) 2				

etc.

by writing

```
      DO 2 I = 1, 10
2     WRITE (3,100) I, (TOTAL(I,J), J = 1, 4)
```

Table 14 indicates permissible array dimensions (i.e., maximum number of
subscripts per variable) in various FORTRAN compilers.

For Review

	Examples
subscript	A(K), A(4), A(K+1), A(2*K), A(2*K−3)
array	A
array element	A(4)
DIMENSION	DIMENSION A(20), B(5,4), C(2,2,5)
dimensionality	
sorting	
interchange	SAVE = X(I)
	X(I) = X(J)
	X(J) = SAVE

For Review	Examples
implied DO loop indexed list	$(X(I), I = 1, N)$
	$((X(I,J), J=1,10),I=1,20)$ $(((X(I,J,K),K=1,3),J=1,2),I=1,4)$ $(X(I,J,K), K = 1, 3)$
double dimension	DIMENSION G(5,8)
triple dimension	DIMENSION H(4,5,3)

EXERCISES

62. Write a program that reads the first three cards of the data deck as a 15-element (single-dimension) array and reprints the values in *reverse* order of reading.

63. The *average deviation* is defined as the arithmetic mean of absolute deviations from an arithmetic mean. That is,

$$\text{A.D.} = \frac{\sum |X - \overline{X}|}{n}$$

Write a program to compute the measure for any data set (maximum 500 items), keypunched one item per card. Use a sentinel card punched 9999. to signal the end of the data deck.

64. Write a program that will read the first nine data items and produce as output the arithmetic means of all possible *different* samples of two items each. Output should be in five columns, showing for each of the 36 samples the integer item numbers (1–9), the two item values, and their mean.

65. Write a program that will read ten values of b and one value of X and compute and print

$$Y = b_1X^9 + b_2X^8 + b_3X^7 + \cdots + b_9X + b_{10}$$

Try to do it in about five executable statements (not including STOP or CALL EXIT).

66. Write a *sorting* program that will rearrange the n elements of array A (read as data) in order of ascending algebraic value so that finally A(1) contains the smallest value and A(n) the largest. Also provide a documentation of the re-

arrangement—that is, an array L that will show the original array position of each value. For example:

Data Order	Output	
3.7	-1.5	2
-1.5	2.0	3
2.0	3.7	1

Test your program on the first 15 data items.

67. Write a program that will read in 20 values of a variable and print the *position numbers* (as integers) of all *pairs* that are *equal* in value.

68. Write a program that *skips* the first three data cards and then reads the next 28 items as a 7-row, 4-column array, keypunched in *column* order (i.e., "vertical" order). Then reprint the array in "horizontal" order (7 rows, 4 columns).

69. Write a program that reads the entire data deck as a 20 × 5 array and then prints as output the column sums.

70. A method used by geologists to measure the degree of similarity between formations uses data arranged as follows:

Characters (0 = no data)	Formation			
	A	B	C	D
I Dolomitic (1 = absent, 2 = present)	2	2	1	0
II Bedding (1 = thin, 2 = thick)	2	1	2	2
III Fossils (1 = absent, 2 = present)	2	2	0	1
IV Iron content (1 = low, 2 = high)	1	2	1	1

The similarity coefficient is defined as

$$S_{Sm} = \frac{m}{n}$$

where m = number of matches
n = number of comparisons

For the data above, the six possible coefficients are:

A	—	—	—	—
B	.50	—	—	—
C	.67	.00	—	—
D	.67	.00	1.00	—
	A	B	C	D

indicating that formations C and D are the most alike, based on available information.

Write a program that will compute the six coefficients for a 4 × 4 matrix. Then generalize it for an i × j matrix, with maximum values of 10 for i and j (using a parameter card to supply dimensionality for each data set). Test both programs by keypunching the data shown above.

71. The *Legendre polynomials* arise in many physical contexts, in electrostatics, acoustics, and quantum mechanics. Write a program that will produce a table of numerical values of Legendre polynomials. The general formula is

$$P_n = \frac{(2n - 1)(P_1)(P_{n-1}) - (n - 1)(P_{n-2})}{n}$$

where

$$P_0 = 1$$

and

$$P_1 = \cos \theta$$

The table should show all values for $\theta = 0°$ to $10°$ in one-degree steps, and in each of these cases for n = 1, 2, 3, 4, 5, and 6. (Convert degrees to radians before using the COS function; multiply degrees by .01745329.) Provide suitable headings and round to *five* decimal places.

72. Write a program that reads and stores the 20 state names and reprints them *alphabetically by column*, as a 4 × 5 array. That is,

ALA.	COL.	FLA.	IND.	LA.
ARIZ.				
ARK.		etc.		
CAL.				

73. For any two-dimensional matrix of observed frequencies (F), chi-square is a statistic computed as

$$\sum \frac{(F - E)^2}{E}$$

where each expected frequency (E) may be computed from

$$E_{ij} = \frac{\sum F_i}{\sum F} (\sum F_j)$$

Write a program to obtain the chi-square value for an m × n matrix (maximum 20 × 20). Read m and n from a parameter card. Test your program on the matrix

	A	B	C
I	6	18	36
II	24	42	54

74. Write a program that reads the data deck and produces as output the state names (columns 76–80), grouped in output segments by first letter, with segments separated by blank lines. For example:

ALA.
ARIZ.
ARK.

CAL.
COL.   (all decisions to be made by the
CONN.   computer, not the programmer)

DEL.
D.C.
                etc.

75. For any two variables X and Y, the *correlation coefficient* may be computed directly, from

$$r = \frac{n \sum XY - \sum X \sum Y}{\sqrt{(n \sum X^2 - (\sum X)^2)(n \sum Y^2 - (\sum Y)^2)}}$$

Write a program that will produce all possible r's for a *matrix* of n variables, each with m observations. (For example, for six variables, $^6C_2 = 15$ possible r values.) Test your program by treating the data deck as five variables, twenty observations each, keypunched as $X_1 - X_1 - X_1 \cdots X_2 - X_2 - X_2 \cdots$, etc.

8 • OTHER CONDITIONAL BRANCH STATEMENTS

We have made extensive use of conditional branching in two forms: directly with the IF statement and indirectly through the DO statement.[1] The conditional branch statement called for by the latter is not explicitly written by the programmer, but is generated in machine language as a comparison of the Index and the limit, at the end of the DO loop range. In this chapter we consider other explicit forms of conditional branch statements.

Computed GO TO

The IF statement we have been using provides up to three alternative routes for the programmer. If more than three alternatives are required, a sequence of IF statements may solve the problem. For example, the following segment permits an execution-time option involving nine alternatives:

```
          ------------------------
          READ (2,10) K
          IF (K − 2) 101, 102, 1
    1     IF (K − 4) 103, 104, 2
    2     IF (K − 6) 105, 106, 3
    3     IF (K − 8) 107, 108, 109
          ------------------------
```

---

[1] Another form, the SENSE SWITCH statement, was mentioned briefly in Chapter 4 and will be referred to later in this chapter.

In this arrangement, the branches reached for various values of K are:

K	Statement Reached
≤ 1	101
2	102
3	103
4	104
5	105
6	106
7	107
8	108
≥ 9	109

The *Computed GO TO* statement is designed to produce this multibranch effect in a single statement:

```
READ (2,10) K
GO TO (101,102,103,104,105,106,107,108,109), K
```

This statement has the effect of nine separate GO TO instructions; the choice between them is conditioned on the current value of an integer variable that must appear to the right of the parentheses. Note that the parentheses contain *statement numbers*, not values of K. Values of K are counted from the left, starting at K = 1. There is no limit to the number of statement numbers (hence, the number of K values) that may be included in the parentheses. The conditioning variable may be any integer variable that has a currently defined value. Serious error results, however, if that value is outside the permissible range, $1 - \#$, where $\#$ is the *number* of statement numbers listed.[2]

Thus the table showing routes for various values of K should be altered to eliminate $\langle$and$\rangle$ for values "1" and "9," when the Computed GO TO is used.

As an example of usage, consider the following program segment, which is designed to form certain sums based on selected values of a subscripted variable (the second, third, fifth, eighth, tenth, thirteenth, and sixteenth values).

---

[2] In many systems, the program is partially destroyed. In some, however, the result is a branch to the next executable statement in sequence. Thus the Computed GO TO is treated as a CONTINUE statement, when its Index is out of permissible range.

```
      ┌DO 1 KOUNT = 1,16
      │GO TO (1,2,2,1,2,1,1,2,1,2,1,2,1,1,2,1,1,2) KOUNT
    2 │SUMX = SUMX + X(KOUNT)
      │SUMX2 = SUMX2 + X(KOUNT)**2
      │SUMX3 = SUMX3 + X(KOUNT)**3
      │SUMX4 = SUMX4 + X(KOUNT)**4
    1 └CONTINUE
```

The Computed GO TO statement is frequently useful in conjunction with an integer variable whose values are computed within the program. For example, consider the following program segment:

```
      L = X/100. + 1.
      GO TO (10,20,30,40,50,60,70,80,90,100), L
```

You should see that these two statements arrange for all the following instructions:

If X is ...	GO TO ...
0 but less than 100	10
100 but less than 200	20
200 but less than 300	30
300 but less than 400	40
400 but less than 500	50
500 but less than 600	60
600 but less than 700	70
700 but less than 800	80
800 but less than 900	90
900 but less than 1000	100

Another programming technique for which the Computed GO TO statement is useful is the treatment of a part of the program as a sort of subprogram, which is to be entered and returned from several times during execution. In the next chapter we discuss several specialized shorthand arrangements available for accomplishing this, which are certainly preferable. The Computed GO

TO statement, however, may be used to construct a programmer-built alternative:

```
            ------------------------
            J = 0
            GO TO 100
    30      -------------------
            -------------------
            -------------------
            -------------------
            GO TO 100
    40      -------------------
            -------------------
            -------------------
            -------------------
            -------------------
            GO TO 100
    50      -------------------
            -------------------
            -------------------
            GO TO 100
    60      -------------------
            -------------------
            -------------------
            -------------------
            GO TO 100
    70      -------------------
            -------------------
            GO TO 100
    80      -------------------
            -------------------
            STOP
    100     -------------------
            -------------------          "subprogram"
            -------------------
            -------------------
            J = J + 1
            GO TO (30,40,50,60,70,80), J
            END
```

This skeletal example illustrates an arrangment for multiple repetition of a program segment, which is thus being treated as a "subprogram." The Computed GO TO statement is used to arrange the return from the repeated routine, conditioned on an integer counter.

Assigned GO TO

Some compilers provide an alternative form of the Computed GO TO statement, which should be avoided by the programmer, for two reasons:

1. It is much less flexible than the Computed GO TO statement, which is also available in these compilers.

2. Since it is absent from many compilers, its use tends to make programs incompatible with other systems.

The Assigned GO TO statement looks like the Computed GO TO statement, with the conditioning variable moved to the left.

GO TO K, (10,20,30,40,50)

The difference, however, is important; in this example, K can only have the following values: 10, 20, 30, 40, or 50 (rather than 1, 2, 3, 4, or 5). Furthermore, K can acquire one of these values *only* through the use of a new statement,

ASSIGN 30 TO K

A side-by-side comparison illustrates the two methods:

Computed GO TO	Assigned GO TO
K = 3	ASSIGN 30 TO K
GO TO (10,20,30,40,50), K	GO TO K, (10,20,30,40,50)

Each of these arrangements branches to statement number 30.

The weakness of the Assigned GO TO arrangement will become obvious if you look back at our four earlier examples of Computed GO TO usage. In the first instance the value of the conditioning variable was determined by reading (as an option parameter), in the second by use of a DO loop Index, and in the third and fourth by computation. *None* of these methods are available for the Assigned GO TO form.

Table 15 shows the availability of Computed GO TO and Assigned GO TO statements in various FORTRAN compilers. (The table also refers to relational and logical operators, discussed in the next section.)

TABLE 15

Conditional GO TO Statements—Relational and Logical Operators

	Computed GO TO		Assigned GO TO		Relational Operators		Logical Operators	
	Yes	No	Yes	No	Yes	No	Yes	No
1[a]	√			√		√		√
2	√		√		√		√	
3	√		√		√		√	
4	√		√		√		√	
5	√		√		√		√	
6	√		√		√		√	
7	√		√			√		√
8	√		√			√		√
9	√		√		√		√	
10	√		√		√		√[b]	
11	√			√	√		√[b]	
12	√		√			√		√
13	√		√		√		√	
14	√		√		√		√	
15	√		√		√		√	
16	√		√			√		√
17	√		√			√		√
18	√			√		√		√
19	√			√		√		√
20	√			√		√		√
21	√		√		√		√	
22	√		√		√		√	
23	√		√		√		√	
24	√		√		√		√	
25	√			√		√		√
26	Not stated		Not stated		√		√	
27	√		√		√		√	
28	√			√		√		√
29	√		√		√		√	
30	√		√			√		√

[a] Compiler number.

[b] Compiler does not permit Logical Variable mode.

TABLE 15 (*continued*)

	Computed GO TO		Assigned GO TO		Relational Operators		Logical Operators	
	Yes	No	Yes	No	Yes	No	Yes	No
31	√		√			√		√
32	√		√			√		√
33	√		√			√		√
34	√		√		√		√	
35	√		√			√		√
36		√	√			√		√
37	√		√		√		√	
38	√		√		√		√	
39	√		√		√		√	
40	√			√		√		√
41	√			√		√		√
42	√		√		√		√	
43	√		√		√		√	
44	√			√		√		√
45	√			√		√		√
46	√		√			√		√
47	√			√	√		√	
48	√			√		√		√
49	√		√			√		√
50	√			√	√			√
51	√			√	√			√
52	√		√		√		√	
53	√		√			√		√
54	√		√			√		√
55	√		√		√		√	
56	√		√		√		√	
57	√		√		√		√	
58	√		√		√		√	
59	√		√			√		√
60	√		√		√		√	
61	√		√		√		√	
62	√		√			√		√
63	√		√		√		√	

TABLE 15 (*continued*)

	Computed GO TO		Assigned GO TO		Relational Operators		Logical Operators	
	Yes	No	Yes	No	Yes	No	Yes	No
64	√		√		√		√	
65	√		√			√		√
66	√		√		√		√	
67	√		√			√		√
68	√		√		√		√	
69	√		√		√		√	
70	√		√		√		√	
71	√		√		√		√	
72	√		√		√		√	
73	√		√		√			√
74	√		√		√		√	
75	√		√		√		√	
76	√		√		√		√	
77	√		√		√		√	
78	√		√		√		√	
79	√		√		√		√	

Logical IF Statement; Relational Operators

The Logical IF statement is misnamed, since it may be used independently of Logical Variables (to be discussed in Chapter 10).[3] It might be better described as a *Verbal IF statement*, since it substitutes abbreviations of verbal relational descriptions for arithmetic operators. The list of such abbreviations follows:

Verbal Meaning	Relational Operator	Equivalent Mathematical Notation
Equal to	.EQ.	$=$
Not equal to	.NE.	$\neq$
Less than	.LT.	$<$
Greater than	.GT.	$>$
Less than or equal to	.LE.	$\leq$
Greater than or equal to	.GE.	$\geq$

---

[3] Even though its *availability* is usually dependent on the availability of the Logical Variable.

The decimal points surrounding each operator are necessary to distinguish it from a possible variable title. These may be used inside IF parentheses in the same manner as *arithmetic* operators; that is, they may separate *any arithmetic expressions*. The phrase constructed lends itself to a *two*-branch alternative, rather than the three permitted by the ordinary arithmetic IF statement. Instead of statement numbers, however, the Logical IF statement itself contains (following the IF brackets) one of the alternative statements, which is executed if the bracket expression is *true* and simply ignored if the bracket expression is *false*. Thus the conditional branch provided by the Verbal IF statement is usually of the triangular form, as shown in the figure.[4] The statement following

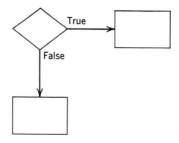

the IF brackets may be any executable statement except another conditional branch statement (or DO statement).

Compare the Arithmetic and Logical versions of the following IF arrangements:

		Arithmetic IF	Logical IF
(1)		IF (X − Y) 1,1,2	IF (X .LE. Y) X = X * 20.
	1	X = X * 20.	DO 3 I = 1,25
	2	DO 3 I = 1,25	
(2)		IF (B − 50.) 3,4,3	IF (B .EQ. 50.) STOP
	3	INCR = INCR + 1	INCR = INCR + 1
		GO TO 2	GO TO 2
	4	STOP	
(3)		IF (K) 6, 7, 7	IF (K .LT. 0.) WRITE (3,100)
	6	WRITE (3,100)	MINT = 3 * K
	7	MINT = 3 * K	

[4] Unless the statement to the right of the IF brackets is a GO TO statement; see example 4.

(4)   8   ----------------   8   ------------------
             ----------------   ------------------
             IF (ANS) 8, 9, 8   IF (ANS .NE. 0.) GO TO 8
      9   WRITE (3,101) ANS   WRITE (3,101) ANS

(5)   IF (3*X−(A+B))110,110,100   IF (3.*X .GT. A+B) X = X/10.
     100   X = X/10.   WRITE (3,I2) X
     110   WRITE (3,12) X

In example 5, note that parentheses surrounding the addition have been dropped in the Logical IF statement. This is possible because *relational operators have lower precedence in execution than arithmetic operators.*

In situations requiring execution of one of *two* alternative statements, rather than the simpler execute/bypass alternatives above, two separate Logical IF statements may be necessary. For example:

	Arithmetic IF	Logical IF
	IF (X(J) − X(K)) I0,11,11	IF (X(J) .GE. X(K)) A = X(K)
10	A = X(J)	IF (X(J) .LT. X(K)) A = X(J)
	GO TO 12	SAVE = X(J)
11	A = X(K)	
12	SAVE = X(J)	

Although the second Logical IF statement may at first appear redundant, you should see that it is necessary to prevent execution of *both* arithmetic statements being treated as alternatives.

As these examples illustrate, the Logical IF statement is a simple substitute for the Arithmetic IF statement, which may frequently save a statement or two (or eliminate statement numbers) and make the program more readable. More importantly, the statements on the right in our examples execute faster than their Arithmetic IF counterparts.

Logical Operators

Most compilers that contain the *relational operators* provide also a set of *logical operators*, which extend further the advantage of Logical over Arithmetic IF statement. These are:

.NOT.
.AND.
.OR.

The logical operators have lower execution precedence than relational operators. Therefore

$$A \text{ .GT. } B \text{ .OR. } C \text{ .LT. } D$$

is executed as though written

$$(A \text{ .GT. } B) \text{ .OR. } (C \text{ .LT. } D)$$

Precedence between logical operators is in the order named above (.NOT. before .AND., .AND. before .OR.). As an example, let us arrange that statement 68 is executed only if A has a value between (and including) 100 and (not including) 200.

Arithmetic IF	Verbal IF
IF (A − 100.) 2,3,3	
3 IF (A − 200.) 68,2,2	
68 COUNT = COUNT + 1.	IF (A .GE. 100. .AND. A .LT. 200.) COUNT = COUNT + 1.
2 ------------------	---------------------

The statement following the Logical IF parentheses is executed only if *both* expressions surrounding .AND. are true. To demonstrate the use of the other two logical operators, let us arrange the same sequence by another method:

$$\text{IF (.NOT. (A .LT. 100. .OR. A .GE. 200.)) COUNT = COUNT + 1.}$$

The ".OR." dictates that the inner parentheses will be ruled *true* if *either* expression is true (i.e., if A is less than 100 or equal to or greater than 200). But if the expression is true, then the A value is out of our specified range. The ".NOT." therefore specifies that the COUNT statement will be executed only if the inner statement is false (i.e., A is in range). If this sounds confusing, a simple paraphrasing of the statement as it reads from left to right should clarify the meaning: "If A is not less than 100 or greater than or equal to 200, then COUNT is to be incremented."

The *relative expressions* used with logical operators need not refer to the same variables. For example,

$$\text{IF (A .GT. B .AND. D .LE. 6.3) GO TO 7}$$

is valid.

Table 15 shows the availability of relational operators and logical operators in various FORTRAN compilers.

External Switches

In Chapter 3 we examined a conditional branch statement that used as a condition the ON-OFF status of an *internal* switch, the "last-card indicator," and also noted that some computers are provided with *program switches* that are *externally* set at the console and may be referred to by FORTRAN conditional branch statements. The purpose of using them is to create execution-time options.

The following segment is designed to let the operator choose between computation with and without transformation to logarithms:

```
              ------------------
              DO 10 K = 1,100
              IF (SENSE SWITCH 2) 20, 10
        20    X(K) = ALOG(X(K))
        10    SUM = SUM + X(K)
              ------------------
```

The statement numbers appear in the order ON, OFF. Thus if program switch 2 is switched ON, the transformation is accomplished by branching to statement 20, while if the switch is left OFF the transformation is bypassed.

As computers have become more proficient at speedy batch processing of jobs stacked sequentially, there has been a tendency to abandon the use of such devices, which slow down the operation while the operator sets the necessary switches. We have examined earlier the possibility of substituting parameter-entry techniques; in the last example, for instance,

```
              ---------------------
              READ (2,11) ICODE
             ┌DO 10 K = 1,100
             │GO TO (20,10), ICODE
        20   │X(K) = ALOG(X(K))
        10   └SUM = SUM + X(K)
              ---------------------
```

If the operator wants the transformation, he punches ICODE as "1"; otherwise it must have the value "2."

In many recent FORTRAN compilers, the "IF" form of external-switch statement has been replaced by a "CALL" statement. (In the next chapter, we explain the programmer's use of "CALL" in writing subprograms.) The usual form of such statements is:

Older Form	Recent Form
IF (SENSE SWITCH 2) 20,10	CALL SSWTCH (2,ICODE)
	GO TO (20,10), ICODE

The number in the parentheses of the CALL statement specifies the switch; the integer variable mentioned will be assigned the value "1" if the specified switch is ON and "2" if it is OFF. Table 16 shows the external switch arrangements available for various FORTRAN compilers.

TABLE 16

External Switches

	CALL SSWTCH	IF (SENSE SWITCH)	Other	None
1[a]				√
2				√
3				√
4	√			
5				√
6				√
7				√
			3 = 1 and 2 6 = 2 and 4	
8		√	5 = 1 and 4 7 = 1, 2, and 4	
9		√		
10				√
11	√			
12		√		
13		√		
14	√			
15	√			
16		√		
17		√		
18				√

[a] Compiler number.

TABLE 16 (*continued*)

	CALL SSWTCH	IF (SENSE SWITCH)	Other	None
19				√
20				√
21				√
22	√			
23				√
24				√
25				√
26				√
27		√		
28				√
29				√
30		√		
31		√		
32		√		
33	√			
34	√			
35		√		
36				√
37	√			
38	√			
39				√
40				√
41				√
42				√
43				√
44			CALL DATSW	
45		√	0 = last card indicator	
46		√		
47	√			
48		√		
49	√		CALL DATSW	
50				√
51	√			
52	√			
53		√		
54		√		

TABLE 16 (*continued*)

	CALL SSWTCH	IF (SENSE SWITCH)	Other	None
55	√			
			CALL SWON	
56	√		CALL SWOFF	
57				√
58				√
59		√		
60				√
61	√			
62		√		
63	√			
64				√
65		√ᵇ		
66	√			
67				√
68	√	√		
69	√	√		
70				√
71	√			
72	√			
73				√
74				√
75	√			
76				√
77				√
78			CALL SWITCH	
79				√

ᵇ Switches set by control card.

Internal Switches

Several conditions that are represented by internal "switch" settings may be of importance to the programmer in various circumstances. *Machine indicator test subroutines* are available in many compilers, which enable the programmer to base branch statements on these conditions. The usual form is the CALL statement.

The programmer may check on whether an arithmetic operation has resulted in overflow or underflow—that is, has produced a numerical result outside the permissible range of (real or integer) storable values.

CALL OVERFL (ITEST)
GO TO (7,8), ITEST

The integer variable named will be set to "1" if an overflow (or underflow) condition exists and to "2" if it does not. (In some compilers, a "3" is used to represent underflow, "1" being reserved for overflow.) An alternative form for some compilers is

IF ACCUMULATOR OVERFLOW 7, 8

If overflow occurs and is not detected by the programmer, the usual result is wrong answers. (Some systems, however, provide console switches that may be set to halt execution if overflow occurs.)

The following program segment makes use of the FORTRAN overflow test, to print a programmer-designed error message when the attempt to compute a geometric mean results in overflow:

```
C     GEOMETRIC MEAN
C     N VALUES—MAX. 100
      DIMENSION X(100)
      READ (2,10) N
      READ (2,11) (X(I)), I = 1, N)
      PROD = 1.
      DO 1 J = 1, N
      PROD = PROD * X(J)
      CALL OVERFL(MESS)
      IF (MESS .EQ. 1) GO TO 2
1     CONTINUE
      FLN = N
      GEOM = PROD**(1./FLN)
      WRITE (3,12) GEOM
      CALL EXIT
2     WRITE (3,13) J
      STOP 99
10    FORMAT (I5)
11    FORMAT (F10.2)
12    FORMAT (17H GEOMETRIC MEAN =,F14.4)
13    FORMAT (17H OVERFLOW ON ITEM,I4)
      END
```

Another internal indicator is ON if an arithmetic expression has resulted in an attempt to divide by zero. Alternative forms of interrogation by the programmer include:

CALL DVCHK(NTEST)   or   IF DIVIDE CHECK 9,10
GO TO (9,10), NTEST

         or   IF QUOTIENT OVERFLOW 9,10

in which, as usual, statement 9 will be executed if the indicator is ON (division by zero having been attempted). The program segment that follows utilizes this indicator to arrange for an alternative computation:

```
     ------------------
13    W = A/(C(1) * C(2) * C(3) * C(4))
      CALL DVCHK(LESS)
      GO TO (15,16), LESS
15   ┌DO 20 K = 1, 4
     │IF (C(K)) 20, 18, 20
18   │C(K) = 1.
20   └CONTINUE
      GO TO 13
16    WRITE (3,102) W
     ------------------
```

Imaginary Switches

Another set of "machine indicator tests" permits the programmer to set an *imaginary* switch ON or OFF and to test this condition at a later point in the program. Two alternative forms currently appear in FORTRAN compilers:

CALL SLITE(4)   or   SENSE LIGHT 4

are statements that turn "ON" the imaginary switch specified (number 4, in this instance). (For most compilers using the statements, CALL SLITE(0) or SENSE LIGHT 0 would turn *all* the imaginary switches *OFF*.) For compilers using the CALL form, the effect of

CALL SLITET (4,K)
GO TO (4,6), K

is to give K the value "1" if the "light" specified is "ON" or "2" if it is "OFF." In the former case, the "light" is then turned OFF—thus K is automatically reset to "2" after each execution of the testing statement. For the SENSE LIGHT version, the switch interrogation and conditional branch are accomplished in a single statement:

IF (SENSE LIGHT 4) 5, 6

with the result of a branch to statement 5 if the "light" is "ON" and to statement 6 if it is "OFF."

To obtain an idea as to what this process may accomplish, as well as to demonstrate a simple programmer-designed substitute, let us examine a program that is designed to rank ("sort") 500 values of a variable, by a technique slightly different from that demonstrated in Chapter 7. Without any imaginary-switch references, the program appears as follows:

```
C       RANKING—METHOD 2A
        DIMENSION X(500)
        READ (2,10) X
       ┌DO 3 K = 1, 499
       │ MAX = 500 − K
       │ DO 3 J = 1, MAX
       │┌IF (X(J) − X(J+1)) 3, 3, 2
    2  ││SAVE = X(J)
       ││X(J) = X(J+1)
       ││X(J+1) = SAVE
    3  └└CONTINUE
        WRITE (3,10) X
        CALL EXIT
   10   FORMAT (8F10.2)
        END
```

In this method, the comparisons called for by the inner loop are made in the order

(1)	(2)	(3)	−−−−−−−etc.
X_1 vs. X_2	X_1 vs. X_2	X_1 vs. X_2	
X_2 vs. X_3	X_2 vs. X_3	X_2 vs. X_3	
X_3 vs. X_4	X_3 vs. X_4	X_3 vs. X_4	
−−−−−−−−−−−	−−−−−−−−−−−	−−−−−−−−−−−	
X_{499} vs. X_{500}	X_{498} vs. X_{499}	X_{497} vs. X_{498}	

TABLE 17

Internal and Imaginary Switches

	CALL OVERFL	CALL DVCHK	CALL SLITE and CALL SLITET	IF ACCUMULATOR OVERFLOW	IF DIVIDE CHECK	IF QUOTIENT OVERFLOW	SENSE LIGHT and IF (SENSE LIGHT)	Other	None
1[a]									✓
2									✓
3									✓
4									
5			✓						
6	✓								✓
7				✓	✓	✓		IF OVERFLOW FAULT	
8				✓	✓	✓		IF DIVIDE FAULT	
9					✓		✓		
10								K = I FALT (i) 0 = OVERFLOW, 1 = DVCHK, 2 = UNDERFLOW	
11		✓	✓					CALL EXFLT (EXPONENT FAULT)	
12							✓	IF OVERFLOW	
13	✓	✓			✓			IF OVERFLOW FAULT	
14		✓	✓				✓	IF DIVIDE FAULT	
15			✓						
16				✓	✓	✓	✓		
17				✓	✓	✓	✓		
18									✓
19									✓
20									✓
21									✓
22	✓		✓						
23									✓
24									✓

25							✓	
26								
27							✓	
28	✓	✓				✓		
29						✓		
30								
31	✓		✓	✓		✓		
32	✓		✓	✓				
33	✓				CALL EDFTST			
34	✓		✓	✓				
35								
36	✓					✓		
37	✓	✓			CALL EOF; CALL PARITY			
38	✓				CALL EOT; CALL REREAD			
39								
40	✓	✓				✓		
41	✓	✓						
42								
43	✓	✓						
44	✓	✓						
45			✓					
46		✓	✓			✓		
47					CALL EOF			
48	✓							
49	✓	✓						
50	✓	✓						
51	✓	✓						
52	✓		✓	✓				
53		✓	✓	✓				
54								

a Compiler number.

TABLE 17 (*continued*)

	CALL OVERFL	CALL DVCHK	CALL SLITE and CALL SLITET	IF ACCUMULATOR OVERFLOW	IF DIVIDE CHECK	IF QUOTIENT OVERFLOW	SENSE LIGHT and IF (SENSE LIGHT)	Other	None
55	✓	✓	✓						
56	✓	✓	✓						
57			✓						✓
58									✓
59							✓		✓
60									✓
61	✓	✓	✓						
62	✓	✓	✓					CALL OVERFLOW	
63	✓	✓	✓				✓		
64	✓	✓	✓						
65	✓	✓	✓	✓	✓				
66	✓	✓	✓	✓		✓	✓		
67	✓								✓
68	✓	✓	✓	✓			✓	IF OVERFLOW / IF FLOATING OVERFLOW	
69	✓	✓	✓	✓			✓	IF OVERFLOW / IF FLOATING OVERFLOW	
70	✓	✓	✓						
71	✓		✓						
72	✓		✓						
73									✓
74									✓
75	✓	✓							
76									✓
77									✓
78	✓	✓	✓	✓	✓	✓	✓		
79									✓

with interchanges in storage being made whenever the left-hand value is higher than the right-hand one.

The first outer-loop execution (1) moves the largest value to the X(500) location, the second (2) moves the next highest to X(499), and so on. The process will completely order all the values (from low to high) after 499 executions of the inner loop.

To shorten average execution time, we shall add some statements that are designed to halt the process (and produce the output) as soon as any run through the inner loop has failed to produce any interchange (indicating that all values are already in order). The four new statements are offset to the right in the version below:

```
C       RANKING—METHOD 2B
        DIMENSION X(500)
        READ (2,10) X
                          INTER = 1
      ⎡DO 3 K = 1, 499
      │                  GO TO (1,4), INTER
      │          1       INTER = 2
      │ MAX = 500 − K
      │⎡DO 3 J = 1, MAX
      ││IF (X(J) − X(J+1)) 3, 3, 2
    2 ││SAVE = X(J)
      ││X(J) = X(J+1)
      ││X(J+1) = SAVE
      ││                 INTER = 1
    3 ⎣⎣CONTINUE
    4   WRITE (3,10) X
        CALL EXIT
   10   FORMAT (8F10.2)
        END
```

The reference variable INTER is set at "2" as the first set of comparisons is begun. You should see that *it is reset to "1" when any interchange of values in storage is performed.* This value of "1" leads to execution of a new set of comparisons, when the Computed GO TO statement is executed. If all the values prove to be in order on any pass through the inner loop, INTER remains at "2," and a branch to the WRITE statement results.

The same procedure is accomplished in the final version by the use of imaginary-switch statements:

```
C      RANKING—METHOD 2C
       DIMENSION X(500)
       READ (2,10) X
                           CALL SLITE(3)           (turns light ON)
      ┌DO 3 K = 1, 499
      │                    CALL SLITET(3,INTER)   (tests light and turns it OFF)
      │                    GO TO (1,4), INTER
  1   │ MAX = 500 − K
      │┌DO 3 J = 1, MAX
      ││IF (X(J) − X(J+1)) 3, 3, 2
  2   ││SAVE = X(J)
      ││X(J) = X(J+1)
      ││X(J+1) = SAVE
      ││                   CALL SLITE(3)           (turns light ON)
  3   └└CONTINUE
  4    WRITE (3,10) X
       CALL EXIT
 10    FORMAT (8F10.2)
       END
```

Additional flexibility for these CALL statements (including the external SSWTCH, as well as SLITE and SLITET) comes from the possibility of using an integer *expression* (containing variables and arithmetic operators), in lieu of the integer constant to represent the switch number. Thus the following are all valid statements:

```
                    CALL SSWTCH (K,ITEST)
                    CALL SLITE (N − 6)
                    CALL SLITET (L*ITEM,INDEX)
```

Table 17 shows availability of, and proper form for, statements referencing internal switches ("machine indicator tests") and imaginary switches ("sense lights") in various FORTRAN compilers.

For Review	Examples
Computed GO TO	GO TO (6,3,4,4,2), K
assign statement	ASSIGN 4 TO K

For Review (*continued*)   **Examples** (*continued*)

Assigned GO TO	GO TO K,(2,3,4,6)
relational operator	.EQ. .NE. .LT. .GT. .LE. .GE.
relative expression	A .LT. B + C
Logical IF statement	IF (A .LT. B + C) A = B + C
logical operator	.NOT. .AND. .OR.
external switches	CALL SSWTCH(2,K)
	GO TO (4,5), K
	IF (SENSE SWITCH 2) 4, 5
internal switches	CALL OVERFL(K)
	GO TO (9,10), K
	IF ACCUMULATOR OVERFLOW 9, 10
	CALL DVCHK(K)
	GO TO (11,12), K
	IF DIVIDE CHECK 11, 12
	IF QUOTIENT OVERFLOW 11, 12
imaginary switches	CALL SLITE(3)
	SENSE LIGHT 3
	CALL SLITET(3,K)
	GO TO (13,14), K
	IF (SENSE LIGHT 3) 13, 14

EXERCISES

76. Write a "compiler" program, using Computed GO TO, which will read, "translate," and execute "statements" written in the following invented language:

Operation	PRACTRAN Code
addition	10
subtraction (2nd operand subtracted from first)	20
multiplication	30
division (1st operand divided by 2nd)	40
exponentiation (2nd operand treated as exponent of 1st)	50
halt	60

Each "statement" card will contain the PRACTRAN code (columns 4, 5) and two operands, with decimal points punched, in columns 11–20 and 21–30. Each such card should generate immediate output of the result of the specified operation. Test your program on the following data:

40	5.	3.
10	5.	3.
50	5.	3.
30	5.	3.
20	5.	3.
60		

77. $\log_e X$ may be obtained from

$$2\left[\frac{X-1}{X+1} + \frac{1}{3}\left(\frac{X-1}{X+1}\right)^3 + \frac{1}{5}\left(\frac{X-1}{X+1}\right)^5 \cdots\right]$$

Write a program that will begin computing $\log_e 1.5$ by this method and will cease the computation when the difference between the result and that returned by the equivalent FORTRAN-supplied function is *less than* .0000001. Output should specify the size of the exponent at this point, as well as showing both computed values. (Use Logical IF, if available.)

78. To solve a common problem in physics, write a program that will read from a parameter card:

$$n = \text{number of resistors}$$

$$\text{KSP} \left\langle \begin{array}{l} 1 = \text{resistors in series} \\ 2 = \text{resistors in parallel} \end{array} \right.$$

and then read from another card

$$R_1, R_2, R_3, \ldots, R_n = \text{resistances}$$
(maximum of 16, keypunched on a single card, in fields of 5)

For resistors in series, compute total resistance:

$$R_t = R_1 + R_2 + R_3 + \cdots + R_n$$

For resistors in parallel, compute total resistance:

$$R_t = \frac{1}{\dfrac{1}{R_1} + \dfrac{1}{R_2} + \dfrac{1}{R_3} + \cdots + \dfrac{1}{R_n}}$$

For the decision, use Logical IF (or Computed GO TO, if your compiler does not provide the relational and logical operators). The program should keep reading data sets until a blank parameter card is encountered. Test your program on two data sets:

$$
\begin{array}{llll}
4 & 1 \\
10 & 20 & 30 & 40 \\
3 & 2 \\
10 & 20 & 10
\end{array}
$$

79. Write a program that will examine all the "external" switches on your computer and print the numbers of those switches that are ON during execution. Label the output,

THE FOLLOWING SWITCHES ARE ON—

80. A program is to read 10 data sets, each containing 10 items. The program must identify by number (1–10) data sets contain *more than one negative* data item. Use *Logical I F* (if available) for the test of negativeness and *imaginary switches* and *Computed GO TO* for the counting and output decision.

81. Rewrite the PRACTRAN program (Exercise 76), so that it uses *external switches*, rather than operation codes appearing as data. That is, any one of the six operations may be called for by setting the appropriate console switch ON; each data card will contain only two real data items (columns 11–20, 21–30). (If your computer has less than six console switches that may be referenced by FORTRAN statements, use *combinations* of switches to make up the deficit.) Test your program on the Exercise 76 data set (arranging for the program to ignore the operation codes).

82. For any set of prices and quantities, *La Speyre's Index* number for each year is computed as

$$
I = \frac{\sum p_n q_o}{\sum p_o q_o}
$$

where p = price
       q = quantity
       n refers to current year
       o refers to *base* year

Write a program that will read p's and q's (in the order p–q–p–q $\cdots$) for up to 20 commodities, for a maximum of 10 years and compute and print La Speyre's Index number for each year. Give the operator the choice of base year, at execution time. Test your program by treating the data deck as a 5-commodity, 10-year set of p's and q's. Let the third year be executed as base year.

83. Write a program that will check your computer's *range* for positive real values, by using any available OVERFLOW test. Arrange for output to show the highest possible nonoverflow value of the base-10 exponent (e.g., shown in Table 6 as ± 38, ± 76, etc.).

84. Write a program to produce an i-period *moving average* (see Exercise 33 for definition) for n items. Let "n" be read from a parameter card; but "i" should be selected by the operator at execution time, by using four console ("external") switches as a set of binary bits—that is, they represent $1 - 2 - 4 - 8$, permitting a maximum $i = 15$ when all four are ON. Test your program with $i = 12$, $n = 20$.

9 · SUBPROGRAM ARRANGEMENTS

We have been making use of several FORTRAN-supplied functions introduced in Chapter 2. Later in this chapter we shall add to our original list other functions provided by some compilers. First, however, we shall examine carefully some methods that enable the programmer to construct his own subprograms.

The principal purpose of *any* subprogram arrangement is avoidance of repetitive programming—a series of computations that is to be repeated may be written once and used many times. The results are savings in programming time, keypunching time, compilation time, and computer storage. In the case of FORTRAN-supplied functions, the writing has been done by the compiler-author for certain computation problems that tend to arise repeatedly in a large variety of problems. The square root function is a good example.

The statement

$$A = SQRT (X + Y) - B$$

is executed as follows:

1. The values of X and Y are looked up in storage and the addition performed.

2. The resulting numerical *argument* is passed to the SQRT subprogram instructions, which produce a new value, the square root of the argument.

3. The computed value is passed back to take the place of SQRT(X + Y), in the *calling statement*.

4. The rest of the statement is executed (look-up of B, subtraction, and placement of result in A storage).

Two methods for duplicating this effect precisely are available in FORTRAN: *statement functions* and *function subprograms*.

Statement Functions

In Chapter 5 we suggested a routine for rounding numbers prior to output, which would work for both positive and negative values. If DELTA is to be printed with two decimal places (e.g., in F10.2), the method was:

$$\text{DELTA} = \text{DELTA} + .005 * (\text{DELTA}/\text{ABS}(\text{DELTA}))$$

suppose that this rounding routine is to be executed several times during the course of a program, for different variables that are to be included in output. The following program contains a *statement function* to accomplish the job:

```
              C     MEAN, VARIANCE, STANDARD DEVIATION
definition →        ROUND(G) = G + .005 * (G/ABS(G))
                    SUMX = 0
                    SUMX2 = 0
                   ┌DO 1 K = 1,200
                   │READ (2,10) X
                   │SUMX = SUMX + X
              1    └SUMX2 = SUMX2 = X * X
                    XMEAN = SUMX/200.
                    XVAR = SUMX2/200. − XMEAN**2
calling            ┌XSTD = ROUND (SQRT(XVAR))
statements         ┤XMEAN = ROUND(XMEAN)
                   └XVAR = ROUND(XVAR)
                    WRITE (3,11) XMEAN, XVAR, XSTD
              10    FORMAT (F10.0)
              11    FORMAT (1H 3F10.2)
                    CALL EXIT
                    END
```

The rules for defining and using such a *statement function* are as follows:

1. The function definition(s) should appear after specification statements (e.g., DIMENSION, REAL), but before the first executable statement of the program. Although this position rule is relaxed in some compilers, the position is acceptable in all.

2. The *left* side of the definition consists of:

(a) An invented title for the function. This title follows all the compiler's rules for titling ordinary variables, as to number of characters, permissible characters, and type implied by first character (unless reversed in an earlier explicit type specification statement),

(*b*) parentheses that surround at least one *dummy argument* (or several dummy arguments separated by commas). Subscripts are not permitted. Note that the "G" in our statement function definition simply indicates that a single real value must be provided by the "calling" statement (in which it also will appear in parentheses, following the function title).

3. The *right* side of the definition consists of any legitimate arithmetic expression, which mentions the arguments bracketed on the left—and shows how they are to be combined to form the required value. This expression may contain FORTRAN-supplied functions or programmer-designed statement functions defined earlier, except that it cannot contain the name of the statement function appearing on the left, that is, your function cannot use itself in computation.

4. Any statement that makes use of the function (a "calling" statement) does so according to the usual rules governing FORTRAN-supplied functions. Thus the function name can appear only on the *right* side of *arithmetic* statements, or within Arithmetic and Logical IF statements. When it appears, it is followed by parentheses that must contain the required arguments, which may be variables, constants, or more complex arithmetic expressions. These arguments must match in *number, order,* and *mode,* but *not necessarily in title,* those in the definition parentheses. These arguments *may* be subscripted, though (as noted earlier) subscripts may not be mentioned in the function definition. They provide the actual values that will be substituted for the dummy variables representing them in the function definition.

The execution of this "calling" statement follows exactly the sequence we have described for the FORTRAN-supplied SQRT function; argument expressions are assigned values, these values are substituted for dummy argument variables in the function definition, the function is evaluated, and the resulting value is passed back to the calling statement.

As an example of the usefulness of additional arguments in the statement function, consider the following *generalized* rounding routine, in which n represents the number of decimal places to be used in output:

$$\text{ROUND(G,N)} = \text{G} + (.5 * .1**\text{N}) * (\text{G/ABS(G)})$$

The added expression produces the following results:

N	$.5(.1)^n$
0	.5
1	.05
2	.005
3	.0005
4	.00005

etc.

This statement function will permit the programmer to specify rounding to any desired decimal place. The calling statement would then appear as follows:

$$FINAL = ROUND(FINAL,4)$$

which calls for rounding of the variable **FINAL**, suitable for output of four decimal digits.

The following examples of statement function definitions and calling statements are all valid:

(1)
```
ROOT(A,B,C) = (−B + SQRT(B**2 − 4. * A * C))/(2. * A)
------------------------------------
PROD = ROOT(X(1), 3.0, W+1.0) * ROOT(X(I), 4.0, W+2. 0)
```

In this example, one root is formed from $A = X_1$, $B = 3.0$, $C = W + 1.0$ and the other from $A = X_1$, $B = 4.0$, $C = W + 2.0$.

(2)
```
ROUND(G,N) = G + (.5 * .1**N) * (G/ABS(G))
PERC(X) = X/SUM * 100.
-------------------------
TRY = ROUND(PERC(CASH),2)
```

Note that SUM is not an argument in the second definition, but is necessary in the computation. Therefore, it must have a defined value when the TRY statement is executed.

(3)
```
NORTH(K,J) = (20 * K)/(J − 10) − 13
-----------------------------
KSPOT = KSPOT + NORTH(KSPOT,M)
```

In this example, the full execution will be as though written

$$KSPOT = KSPOT + ((20 * KSPOT)/(M - 10) - 13)$$

(4)
$$Z(R) = .5 * (ALOG(1. + R) - ALOG(1. - R))$$

$$TRANS = Z(PM/(SX*SY))$$

Statistics students may recognize that the calling statement results in (a) computation of the correlation coefficient, by the product-moment method, and (b) transformation to Fisher's Z value.

Function Subprograms

The statement function is useful only for computations that can be performed in a single statement. Furthermore, it can generate only one value to be returned to the calling statement.

With regard to the first of these limitations, consider a routine designed to produce factorial n (n! = 1*2*3*4 ··· *n):

```
        FACT = 1.0
       ┌DO 1000 K = 1,N
       │FN = K
 1000  └FACT = FACT * FN
```

This segment is converted to proper form for a *function subprogram* simply by adding three statements:

```
        FUNCTION FACT(N)
        FACT = 1.0
       ┌DO 1000 K = 1,N
       │FN = K
 1000  └FACT = FACT * FN
        RETURN
        END
```

The FUNCTION statement identifies what follows as a *function subprogram*; as in the case of the statement function, this identification prohibits execution of the following statements until and unless called for by a *main program*. That is, these statements merely *define* the function. The invented title and the dummy argument(s) appear after the word "FUNCTION," following the same construction rules as for statement functions. The title variable must be mentioned at least once on the left side of an arithmetic statement in the subprogram,[1] since it must acquire a value to return to the calling program.

The RETURN statement is a branch statement that returns control to the calling statement (in the main program) that mentioned the function name. A function subprogram may contain more than one RETURN statement (we shall show such an example shortly).

The use of the END statement, which is mandatory, signifies one of the most interesting features of the function subprogram: it is treated by the compiler as a completely separate program and may be so treated by the programmer. Once written, therefore, it may be used in conjunction with several (or many) main programs. This extends the avoidance of repetitive programming to a new dimension, as some of our examples will illustrate. It also suggests that a function that may be useful in more than one program should be written as a function subprogram, even though it might be done as a statement function. Thus:

```
FUNCTION ROUND (G,N)
ROUND = G + (.5 * .1 ** N) * (G/ABS(G))
RETURN
END
```

This makes the ROUND function available in all (calling) programs, though it now should not be written into any of them.

Let us make use of the factorial-number function subprogram in a program to evaluate the *combinations* formula,

$$^{n}C_{r} = \frac{n!}{r!(n-r)!}$$

(number of combinations of n things taken r at a time; also written $\left(\dfrac{n}{r}\right)$).

```
        COMBINATIONS
        READ (2,10) N, IR
        COMB = FACT(N)/(FACT(IR)*FACT(N−IR))
        WRITE (3,11) COMB
        STOP
1       FORMAT (2I5)
11      FORMAT (1H F10.0,13H COMBINATIONS)
        END
```

---

[1] The only exception to this is the possibility of mentioning it in an input list within the subprogram.

The main program and subprogram(s) may be compiled independently; but any subprograms referenced must be available as object programs[2] when the main program is executed. The prior availability of the FACT function makes the COMBINATIONS program extremely simple to write.

Let us take the idea a step further, by converting the COMBINATIONS program to a separate function subprogram:

```
FUNCTION COMB(N,IR)
COMB = FACT(N)/(FACT(IR)*FACT(N−IR))
RETURN
END
```

We have removed input and output statements and FORMAT, since our intention is to use the subprogram in conjunction with main programs that will perform the input/output activities. Note that the use of "N" in both subprograms does not create conflict (though we will load both together, since one calls the other); all arguments mentioned as dummies may be duplicated in other subprograms or in the main program, without causing error. The same is true for *all* variable names in the subprogram (including those not used as arguments) and also for all *statement numbers* used.

The binomial expansion

$$(q + p)^n$$

has $(n + 1)$ terms, designated as terms $0, 1, 2, 3, 4, \ldots, n$. The rth term is computed

$$^nC_r \ p^r \ q^{n-r}$$

A program to compute all the terms[3] of the binomial may now be written as follows:

```
C       BINOMIAL TERMS
        READ (2,10) P, Q, N
        NUM = N + 1
       ⌈DO 1 M = 1, NUM
       │ K = M− 1
       │ TERM = COMB(N,K)*P**K*Q**(N−K)
1      ⌊WRITE (3,11) K, TERM
10      FORMAT (2F10.4,I5)
11      FORMAT (I6,F14.4)
        CALL EXIT
        END
```

---

[2] Methods for storing them are discussed in Chapter 12.

[3] The terms of the binomial may be obtained more efficiently, however, by taking advantage of the fact that the rth term may be built up from the $(r − 1)$th term.

The two subprograms must be available in secondary storage (e.g., disk, tape; see Chapter 12) or loaded along with the main program:

```
C        FACTORIAL SUBPROGRAM
         FUNCTION FACT(N)
         FACT = 1.0
        ⎡DO 1000 K = 1, N
        ⎢FN = K
1000    ⎣FACT = FACT * FN
         RETURN
         END


C        COMBINATIONS SUBPROGRAM
         FUNCTION COMB(N,IR)
         COMB = FACT(N)/(FACT(IR)*FACT(N−IR))
         RETURN
         END
```

The most significant result of this programming effort is availability as part of a permanent library of functions of the COMB and FACT subprograms. Building a library of such subprograms becomes a key activity at every computer installation.

An example of a function subprogram with more than one RETURN statement follows:

```
         FUNCTION RATIO(X,Y)
         IF (X − Y) 100, 100, 101
100      RATIO = X/Y
         RETURN
101      RATIO = Y/X
         RETURN
         END
```

The function is designed to return to the main program the ratio of any two real arguments, using the smaller as the numerator. A calling statement might read,

```
         ANS = RATIO(A,B) * SUM
```

Subscripted Variables in Subprograms

Function subprograms cannot mention subscripts in the list of dummy arguments. However, the variables mentioned *may* be array names, in which case a DIMENSION statement (or a type specification statement containing dimension information) must appear in the subprogram. *This DIMENSION statement will not have the usual effect of reserving storage locations.* No subprogram dummy argument actually receives an assigned storage location during compilation, since the main program that supplies the actual arguments (in a calling statement) will also have provided their storage locations (passing proper addresses to the subprogram). Thus the DIMENSION statement in the subprogram is used only to indicate that the dummy variable is to be treated as an array in main programs calling the subprogram. A common practice is to write (1) in the subprogram DIMENSION statement when a dummy argument is declared.

Let us demonstrate by writing a function subprogram that will compute the arithmetic mean of the first n values in a real array.

FUNCTION MEAN(X,N)

is not a good beginning, for the function title "MEAN" implies integer mode. This is not desirable, since arithmetic means frequently have decimal content. The implicit mode of the function title variable may be overridden by an "instant" explicit type specification; for example, we might try

REAL FUNCTION MEAN(X,N)

However, this is dangerous, since any main program using the function would have to specify

REAL MEAN

in order that the returned value could be properly interpreted. Function subprogram titles are more safely left to implicit type specification. (This is why the FORTRAN-supplied logarithm function name is ALOG, not LOG.) Therefore, we shall use "XMEAN" as the function title. The entire subprogram looks like this:

```
        FUNCTION XMEAN(X,N)
        DIMENSION X(1)
        SUMX = 0
       ┌DO 1 K = 1,N
     1  └SUMX = SUMX + X(K)
        FN = N
        XMEAN = SUMX/FN
        RETURN
        END
```

The values of a real subscripted variable, and the value of the integer parameter, must be supplied by the calling program. This is accomplished, as usual, by mention in a calling statement that contains the function title and bracketed arguments. The array name appears *without* subscript information, to indicate the entire dimensioned array. (But note that if the parameter argument used is less than the true array size, our subprogram will compute the mean of the first n elements.) The following main program segment uses the subprogram to compute the ratio of two means:

```
          DIMENSION A(40), B(80)
          READ (2,10) A, B
   10     FORMAT (8F10.4)
          RATIO = XMEAN(A,40)/XMEAN(B,80)
          _____

          _____
```

The subprogram is called twice. On the first call, "A" is recognized as the dummy "X" and "40" is in correct position (and mode) to substitute for the dummy "N"; on the second call, "B" values and "80" are used by the subprogram.

"Adjustable Dimensions"

A method is available in some compilers (see Table 18) for making the subprogram DIMENSION size "adjustable." This is done by writing the subprogram DIMENSION statement in a manner that would be illegal in the main program—by using an integer *variable*, which must be mentioned as an argument in the FUNCTION definition and calling statements and thus passed as a value from the main program. In our example (the XMEAN function), since N is already mentioned as a definition argument and has the proper meaning, the subprogram statement may be rewritten

DIMENSION X(N)

This device appears rather redundant, however, since we have illustrated that the compiler's nonstorage reaction to subprogram DIMENSION statements *for dummy arguments* makes the array size effectively adjustable at all times (even if an integer constant is used). That is, the main program DIMENSION statement actually dictates the size of the array mentioned in any calling statement. Nor could the "adjustable DIMENSION" feature be used for nonargument variables, since these must be provided with reserved storage by the subprogram. For example,

```
FUNCTION TRY(Q,N)
DIMENSION Q(20), R(10)
```

has the effect during compilation of reserving ten locations for R, but none for Q. Therefore,

```
DIMENSION Q(N), R(N)
```

would not be accepted by compilers offering the "adjustable DIMENSION" feature, since locations for R values could not be properly allocated.

```
DIMENSION Q(N), R(10)
```

would be acceptable, but

```
DIMENSION Q(1), R(10)
```

would have the same effect.

When a dummy argument is to be declared as a *multidimensional* array, however, the variable DIMENSION possibility becomes more useful. For

```
FUNCTION DIAG(W)
DIMENSION W(1,1)
```

will *not* work properly; individual elements of the two-dimensional array cannot be properly located when mentioned in a subprogram using this technique. For example, the storage address (relative to the beginning address for the array) of

$$W(2,2)$$

will be different for a 2×3 and a 3×4 matrix:

Since internal storage is in column order, the (2, 2) element is the *fourth* stored value in the smaller array and the *fifth* in the larger. In this situation,

```
FUNCTION DIAG(W,M,N)
DIMENSION W(M,N)
```

will permit use of the subprogram with main programs containing arrays of assorted sizes.

As an alternative, however, we may observe that *constants* representing *maximum* values of m and n may be used in both subprogram and all calling programs, to accomplish the same effect (at a cost of some wasted storage). Thus

```
FUNCTION DIAG(W,M,N)
DIMENSION W(20,20)
```

will work for all main programs containing the same array size *declaration*; part of the reserved storage will usually be empty. (M and N are retained as arguments, to serve as DO statement limits, in the subprogram.) A calling program using a 12 × 6 matrix might be written,

```
DIMENSION X(20,20)
READ (2,10) ((X(I,J), J = 1, 6), I = 1, 12)
- - - - - - - - - - - - - - - - - - - - 
FIRST = 3.0 * DIAG(X,12,6)
- - - - - - - - - - - - - - - - - - - - 
```

Thus the proper technique for writing DIMENSION statements, when the compiler lacks the adjustable-DIMENSION feature and a subprogram argument is to be a multidimensional array, is as follows:

1. Mention the dimensions as variables in the subprogram argument list and as variables, constants, or other expressions in the calling statement argument list, just as would be done with adjustable DIMENSION available.

2. In the DIMENSION statements, use integer constants specifying *maximum* array dimensions, which must be the same for both subprogram(s) and main program.

Subroutine Subprograms

There is a weakness shared by both the statement function and the function subprogram; each can (and must) return only a single value to the calling statement. It would be convenient, for example, to have a single subprogram that could provide both *arithmetic mean* and *standard deviation*. We have seen that function subprograms may *call* other function subprograms, so that a separate function for the standard deviation might *make use* of our XMEAN function, just as it calls the compiler-supplied SQRT:

```
          FUNCTION STDEV(A,K)
          DIMENSION A(1)
          XBAR = XMEAN(A,K)
          SUM = 0
         ⌈DO 1 L = 1, K
    1     ⌊SUM = SUM + (A(L) − XBAR)**2
          FK = K
          STDEV = SQRT(SUM/FK)
          RETURN
          END
```

A main-program calling statement using both functions could then say,

$$\text{HIGH} = \text{XMEAN(OBS,NUM)} + 2.576 * \text{STDEV(OBS,NUM)}/\text{SQRT(F}-1.)$$

During execution of this statement the XMEAN subprogram will actually be used twice, first returning a value to the main program and then the same value to the STDEV subprogram. Therefore, the statement calls for three executions of two subprograms.

We may note that a function subprogram can *produce* more than a single value, if by "produce" we mean merely compute and output:

```
          FUNCTION XMEAN(X,N)
          DIMENSION X(1)
          SUMX = 0.
          SUMX2 = 0.
         ⌈DO 1 L = 1, N
         |SUMX = SUMX + X(L)
    1     ⌊SUMX2 = SUMX2 + X(L)**2
          FN = N
          XMEAN = SUMX/FN
          STDEV = SQRT(SUMX2/FN − XMEAN**2)
          WRITE (3,15) STDEV
   15     FORMAT (11H ST. DEV. =,F15.5)
          RETURN
          END
```

Even though in this way the standard deviation will be *recorded* (on an output record), it *cannot* be made available, by this technique, to the main program that calls the function.

The problem is solved by the *subroutine subprogram* form. In our last subprogram, we merely substitute for the FUNCTION definition statement,

SUBROUTINE MSTD(X,N,XMEAN,STDEV)

and extract the WRITE and FORMAT statements, which are no longer needed. The mention of XMEAN and STDEV in the argument list makes both of those computed values available to the main program, which will also mention two real arguments in the same position in calling statements.

The rules that govern use of this new subprogram type are:

1. The invented title of a *subroutine subprogram* is used *only* as a title and does not acquire a value during the computation. Thus the name MSTD has no storage location allocated to it.

2. The first character of the invented title does not dictate a mode (real or integer), since the title is not used as a variable. The title need not appear on the left side of any arithmetic statement in the subprogram (as the FUNCTION title *must*).

3. Dummy arguments may be mentioned on the left side of arithmetic statements in the subprogram. This "redefinition" of arguments is prohibited in function subprograms. This permits the programmer to include in the argument list not only variables whose values are to be passed from main program to subprogram, but also those whose values are to be computed *by* the subprogram and passed to the main program. All values that are to be passed *in either direction* are listed as arguments.[4]

4. The calling statement is of the form

CALL MSTD(OBS,NUM,XBAR,SX)

As usual, the arguments may be represented as variables, constants, or other valid arithmetic expressions, including those using functions. To this list we add the "Hollerith constant" mentioned in Chapter 6, which is available in some compilers (see Table 27, Chapter 11). A usage example appears at the end of this section.

The calling statement shown lists as arguments two variables whose values are passed to the subprogram for use in computation and two variables whose

---

[4] Unless the COMMON statement is used. This will be discussed shortly. Some FORTRAN compilers permit the inclusion of "extra" arguments in *function* subprogram definitions, for return of more than one value to the calling program. For these compilers, paragraph 3 above describes both types of subprogram; and our original problem could be solved by

FUNCTION XMEAN(X,N,STDEV)

values are *computed* by the subprogram and passed back to the calling program. That is, X and N (OBS, NUM) are both mentioned to the *right* of equal-signs in the subprogram, while XMEAN and STDEV (XBAR, SX) are each defined on the *left* of an equal-sign. Note that XBAR and SX will not be declared as undefined variables when the main program is compiled, even though their first mention occurs in the CALL statement.

Since there is no limit to the number of arguments that may appear in the definition and calling statements (so long as they match in number, order, and mode), the subroutine subprogram can return an unlimited number of values to the main program that calls it.

5. Instead of returning to the *calling statement* with a value for the subroutine title variable, the subroutine subprogram returns control to the first executable statement *following* the CALL statement. It does not return any value for the title variable; but all the argument values are available.

To review these points, compare our RATIO subprogram in its original FUNCTION form with the same operation written as a subroutine subprogram:

	Function Subprogram		Subroutine Subprogram
	FUNCTION RATIO(X,Y)		SUBROUTINE RATIO(X,Y,R)
	IF (X − Y) 100, 100, 101		IF (X − Y) 100, 100, 101
100	RATIO = X/Y	100	R = X/Y
	RETURN		RETURN
101	RATIO = Y/X	101	R = Y/X
	RETURN		RETURN
	END		END

And in the calling program,

	ANS = RATIO(A,B)		CALL RATIO(A,B,ANS)

In the FUNCTION version, the ratio is computed in a statement that uses the FUNCTION title (RATIO) as storage location and is returned to the calling statement, which has also mentioned the title, before the actual arguments. In the SUBROUTINE version, the ratio is computed as R, which is a subprogram *argument*, and is returned to the main program as ANS, an argument appearing in proper position in the CALL statement. The subprogram title is mentioned in the CALL statement, but is not used in either program to store a value.

As the comparison illustrates, many subprograms might be written in either form. The choice between *function subprogram* and *subroutine subprogram*

is usually decided in favor of the former when only a single value is to be
returned. They are alike in all usage rules except the few we have distinguished,
with one more exception: a subroutine subprogram may be written *without*
dummy arguments (in which case, of course, the calling statement can have no
arguments). This arrangement usually signifies, however, that no values will
be passed from main program to subprogram *or* from subprogram to main
program.[5] In some instances, this is because the subprogram has its own input
and/or output statements. For example, the following subprogram is designed
to print an error message, for any main program that is checking sequence
numbers on cards, as data are read in:

```
       SUBROUTINE ERROR
       WRITE (1,1001)
1001   FORMAT (25HDATA CARD OUT OF SEQUENCE)
       RETURN
       END
```

A segment of a calling program might read:

```
       -----------------
       DO 1 K = 1, N
       READ (2,10) NUM, A, B, C, D
       IF (NUM .NE. K) CALL ERROR
       -----------------
       -----------------
```

In this example, however, the error message does not seem overly helpful; the
addition of an argument may improve its usefulness:

```
       SUBROUTINE ERROR(MISS)
       WRITE (1,1001) MISS
1001   FORMAT (35HDATA CARD OUT OF SEQUENCE AFTER NO.,I5)
       RETURN
       END
```

And the calling statement would specify:

```
       IF (NUM .NE. K) CALL ERROR(K−1)
```

The *Hollerith constant* (see Table 25) may be used as an argument when the
subprogram is to produce output in "A" FORMAT. For example,

---

[5] Unless the COMMON statement is used. See the next section.

```
          SUBROUTINE FINISH(NAME)
          WRITE (3,10) NAME
    10    FORMAT (' EXECUTION OF', A6, 'COMPLETE')
          RETURN
          END
```

The FORMAT statement employs *literal transfer* for alphameric output of three "fixed" words and A FORMAT for output of the main program name, transmitted to the subprogram as a Hollerith constant. The calling statement specifies the Hollerith constant by using the nH alphameric notation:

```
          CALL FINISH (6HUPDATE)
```

The COMMON Statement

The COMMON statement is a convenient method for passing values between main program and subprograms *without mentioning them as arguments*. It is a *specification* statement—used during compilation rather than execution, just as DIMENSION, REAL, and INTEGER are used. Use of the statement in our SUBROUTINE RATIO subprogram removes all arguments from the subprogram definition and from calling statements, without altering the results:

Without COMMON	With COMMON
```SUBROUTINE RATIO(X,Y,R)```	```SUBROUTINE RATIO```
```IF (X − Y) 100, 100, 101```	```COMMON X,Y,R```
```100 R = X/Y```	```IF (X − Y) 100, 100, 101```
```RETURN```	```100 R = X/Y```
```101 R = Y/X```	```RETURN```
```RETURN```	```101 R = Y/X```
```END```	```RETURN```
	```END```

In the calling program,

```
                              COMMON A, B, ANS
                              ----------------
          CALL RATIO(A,B,ANS)  CALL RATIO
```

We have noted that the dummy arguments mentioned in a subprogram do not have to agree in *title* with arguments used in a calling statement within the

main program. This applies also to variables mentioned in COMMON statements. As usual, the variables should agree between programs as to *number*,
order, and *mode*. Thus

        SUBROUTINE FORM   (subprogram)
        COMMON A, B, C, K
        ————————————————

in conjunction with

        COMMON X, Y, Z, J   (main program)
        ————————————————
        CALL FORM

creates equivalence between three pairs of real variables and one pair of integer
variables. That is, a total of only four storage locations (three real and one
integer) will be used.

It may be useful to outline the actual method employed by the compiler,
in arranging the storage. In reaction to the COMMON statement, it reserves
storage for the accompanying list of variables in a special area of storage (the
"COMMON area"), in the order in which they are named. Since this reaction
is the same whenever the statement is encountered (including subprogram com-
pilations), and the compiler always begins the reservations at the beginning of
the COMMON area, X and A in our example are stored in the same location
(which can now be reached by either reference title) as are Y and B, Z and C,
and J and K. (Obviously, the modes of the variables so listed must match
"vertically"—that is, between programs.)

The important result of using the COMMON statement should be stressed:
subprograms and calling statements need not (in fact, *cannot*) mention as
arguments variables whose values are to be passed from main program to subprogram (or vice versa), if these are listed in COMMON statements in both
programs.[6] For example, consider the subprogram

        SUBROUTINE PROD   (subprogram)
        COMMON F, G, H
        H = F * G
        RETURN
        END

_____

[6] Except that *function subprograms* must mention at least one argument, which must
also appear in the calling statement.

The two real values to be supplied by the main program, and the computed value to be returned, need not be listed as arguments, for:

```
        COMMON R, S, T                          (main program)
        READ (2,10) R, S
        CALL PROD
        WRITE (3,10) T
        CALL EXIT
10      FORMAT (1H 2F10.2)
        END
```

When the subprogram is called, the values of "F" and "G" are in storage, having been read in as "R" and "S" and placed in the first two COMMON area locations. Similarly, when the calling program mentions "T," the location is already filled with the value computed by the subprogram as "H" and located in the third position of the COMMON area storage. If the COMMON statements were not used, however, the T location would be empty unless H were mentioned as an argument in the SUBROUTINE statement and T mentioned as an argument in the CALL statement.

When *subscripted* variables are to be placed in COMMON storage for passage between programs, two methods of handling DIMENSION and COMMON are available to the programmer:

```
either          SUBROUTINE CALC
                COMMON X(25)

or              SUBROUTINE CALC
                DIMENSION X(25)
                COMMON X
```

The first method combines the function of COMMON and DIMENSION, eliminating the need for (and rendering invalid) any mention of X in a DIMEN-SION statement. The second method uses the DIMENSION statement, in which case the subscript information must be omitted from the COMMON statement that follows[7] (and which implicitly refers to the entire array). This follows the general rule, established in Chapter 7 in relation to explicit type statements, that dimension information should appear in the *earliest* specification statement mentioning the variable and should not be repeated thereafter.

Note that in either method the subprogram must provide a genuine

---

[7] Most compilers require that DIMENSION statements precede COMMON statements, when both are used. Order of specification statements is discussed in Chapter 11.

number for the dimensionality, since COMMON storage *is* reserved by the subprogram (i.e., actual storage location addresses are set aside, noted, and referenced with names). The "adjustable DIMENSION" feature cannot be applied to COMMON statements for this reason.

Labeled COMMON

Many compilers permit the division (as directed by the programmer) of the COMMON storage area into separate "labeled" sections. The insertion of the label that names and identifies as separate a COMMON area is accomplished by enclosing it between slashes. Thus

COMMON /FIRST/A,B,C/LAST/D,E

establishes two labeled areas. If an unlabeled (*blank COMMON*) area is to be included, it may appear at the first part of the statement without slashes, *or* be preceded by two consecutive slashes, anywhere in the statement:

COMMON DELTA, CROSS/FIRST/A,B,C/LAST/D,E

or   COMMON /FIRST/A,B,C//DELTA,CROSS/LAST/D,E

are equivalent.

This division into one blank and two labeled areas of COMMON storage would permit the programmer to specify equivalences (i.e., shared storage) in an order other than that originally used. For example, another COMMON statement in the same program could insert variables F and G in the "LAST" area merely by writing

COMMON/LAST/F,G

If this statement were written instead as

COMMON F,G

the new variables would follow DELTA and CROSS in the blank COMMON area.

Be warned that the usefulness of *labeled COMMON* is limited to highly specialized situations. In many instances, the programmer using the method realizes post facto that removal of all the "labels" does not change the execution of his programs.

Suppose that the statement

COMMON/LAST/F,G

appeared in a *subprogram*, when the *main program* contains our earlier statement

COMMON DELTA,CROSS/FIRST/A,B,C/LAST,D,E

Then shared storage has been established between D and F and between E and G. But we must observe that the same effect would be accomplished with

main program

COMMON D,E,DELTA,CROSS,A,B,C

subprogram

COMMON F,G

Usefulness of *labeled common* is more probable (though it is not indispensable) when more than two programs are to share common storage. For instance, suppose that two subprograms are in storage, each containing a different COMMON arrangement:

1st subprogram

COMMON X(100)

2nd subprogram

COMMON W(15,5)

Now a main program is to be written that calls *both* of the subprograms, passing 100 values to the first and 75 completely different values to the second. A solution not using labeled COMMON would require COMMON statements with matching total storage length in the three programs:

1st subprogram

COMMON X(100), DUMMY(15,5)

2nd subprogram

    COMMON DUMMY(100),W(15,5)

main program

    COMMON RATE(100),PRICE(15,5)

However, if the subroutine program COMMON statements had originally been written with labels, they would not require changing, for:

1st subprogram

    COMMON /S1/X(100)

2nd subprogram

    COMMON/S2/W(15,5)

main program

    COMMON /S1/RATE(100)/S2/PRICE(15,5)

The EXTERNAL Statement

We have indicated that the arguments mentioned in calling statements may be variables (with or without subscripts), constants, or more complicated arithmetic expressions. One further possibility is permitted: the use of a function name as an argument. When this is done, the main program must have an EXTERNAL statement, which specifies that this argument is to be found outside both main program and subprogram. For example,

```
C    FUNCTION SUBPROGRAM TO OBTAIN RECIPROCALS OF CERTAIN
C    FUNCTIONS OF D
     FUNCTION RECIP(D,F)
     RECIP = 1./F(D)
     RETURN
     END

C    THIS IS THE CALLING PROGRAM
     EXTERNAL SQRT, ALOG
     ----------------------
     RSQRT = RECIP(X,SQRT)
     RLOG = RECIP(X,ALOG)
     ----------------------
```

The ENTRY Statement

Occasionally the programmer wishes to provide different points of entry into a subprogram, which may be distinguished by differences in the CALL statement. For example,

```
C     SUBPROGRAM TO COMPUTE ARITHMETIC AND/OR GEOMETRIC MEAN
      SUBROUTINE MEANS(N)
      COMMON X(100),XA,XG
      SUM = 0.0
     ┌DO 1000 K = 1,N
1000 └SUM = SUM + X(K)
      FN = N
      XA = SUM/FN
      ENTRY GEOM(N)
      PROD = 1.0
     ┌DO 1001 K = 1, N
1001 └PROD = PROD * X(K)
      FN = N
      XG = PROD**(1./FN)
      RETURN
      END
```

If the programmer wants *both* arithmetic and geometric mean, the main program calling statement is

$$\text{CALL MEANS(K)}$$

This enters the subprogram at its first executable statement (SUM = 0.0). Since ENTRY is a nonexecutable statement, it is ignored when encountered during this execution of the subprogram.

For geometric mean only, the calling statement would read,

$$\text{CALL GEOM(K)}$$

A Programmer-Supplied Function

In the next section we add to our original list of (the most common) FORTRAN-supplied functions. Some of these are designed to select the largest or smallest of a number of arguments. As a review in transition, let us write something similar as a function subprogram. The routine is designed to select the largest value of a subscripted variable (i.e., largest element of a one-dimensional array).

```
FUNCTION BIG(N)
COMMON X(300)
BIG = X(1)
DO 1002 K = 2,N
IF (BIG .LT. X(K)) BIG = X(K)
1002  CONTINUE
RETURN
END
```

In the calling program,

```
COMMON W(300)
READ (2,10) (W(K),K=1,50)
A = BIG(50)

_____

_____
```

We noted earlier that an array mentioned in a COMMON statement *cannot* have adjustable dimensions, that is, COMMON X(N) would not be legal. However, the use of the COMMON arrangement in this example limits the required storage to 300 locations, regardless of the number appearing (maximum 300) in the calling program.

TABLE 18

Subprograms and Related Statements

	Statement Functions	Function Subprograms	Subroutine Subprograms	Adjustable Dimensions	COMMON Blank	COMMON Labeled	External	Entry
1[a]	√	√	√		√			
2	√	√	√	√	√	√	√	
3	√	√	√	√	√	√	√	
4	√	√	√	√	√	√	√	
5		√	√	√	√	√	√	√
6		√	√		√	√		
7			√					
8			√		√			
9	√	√	√	√	√	√	√	√
10	√	√	√		√	√	√	
11		√	√		√		√	√
12	√	√	√		√		√	

[a] Compiler number.

TABLE 18 (*continued*)

	Statement Functions	Function Subprograms	Subroutine Subprograms	Adjustable Dimensions	COMMON Blank	COMMON Labeled	External	Entry
13	√	√	√	√	√	√	√	√
14	√	√	√	√	√	√	√	√
15	√	√	√	√	√	√	√	√
16	√	√	√		√		F	
17	√	√	√		√			
18	√	√	√		√			
19								
20								
21	√	√	√		√	√	√	
22	√	√	√	√	√	√	√	
23	√	√	√	√	√	√	√	
24	√	√	√	√	√	√	√	
25		√	√	√	√			
26	√	√	√		√	√	√	
27	√	√	√	√	√		F	
28		√	√		√			
29	√	√	√	√	√	√	√	√
30		√	√		√	√b	√	
31	√	√	√		√		F	
32		√	√		√			
33	√	√	√		√		√	
34	√	√	√	√	√	√	√	√
35	√	√	√		√			
36	√	√	√		√		√	√
37	√	√	√		√	√	√	
38	√	√	√		√	√	√	
39	√	√	√	√	√	√	√	√
40	√	√	√		√		√	
41	√	√	√		√			
42	√	√	√	√	√	√	√	√
43	√	√	√	√	√	√	√	√
44	√	√	√		√		√	
45	[In auto-coder only]							
46	√	√	√		√			
47		√	√	√	√		√	
48								

b Restricted to one-letter names.

TABLE 18 (*continued*)

	Statement Functions	Function Subprograms	Subroutine Subprograms	Adjustable Dimensions	COMMON Blank	COMMON Labeled	External	Entry
49	√	√	√		√		√	
50	√	√	√		√		√	
51		√	√		√			
52	√	√	√	√	√	√	√	
53	√	√	√		√			
54	√			In main program				
55	√	√	√	√	√	√	√	√
56	√	√	√	√	√	√	√	
57	√	√	√	√	√			
58	√	√	√	√	√			
59	√	√	√		√		√	
60	√	√	√	√	√	√	√	
61	√	√	√	√	√	√	√	
62	√	√	√		√			
63	√	√	√	√	√	√	√	√
64	√	√	√		√	√	√	√
65	√	√	√		√			
66	√	√	√	√	√	√	√	
67	√	√	√		√		√	
68	√	√	√	√	√	√	√	
69	√	√	√	√	√	√	√	√
70	√	√	√	√	√	√	√	√
71	√	√	√	√	√	√	√	
72	√	√	√	√	√	√	√	
73	√	√	√	√	√	√	√	
74	√	√	√	√	√	√	√	
75		√	√		√	√	√	
76	√	√	√	√	√	√	√	
77	√ c	√	√	√	√	√	√	√
78	√	√	√	√	√	√	√	
79	√	√	√	√	√	√	√	

c Needs "DEFINE" statement.

Table 18 shows availability of the three forms of programmer-supplied subprogram arrangements and related statements.

FORTRAN-Supplied Functions

The eight functions listed in Chapter 2 are found in most FORTRAN compilers. Those discussed below vary from rare to frequent inclusion in basic compilers.

Trigonometric Functions

In addition to SIN, COS, and ATAN, mentioned earlier, we now list:

TAN(A)	tangent of a
TANH(A)	hyperbolic tangent of a
COTAN(A)	cotangent of a
SINH(A)	hyperbolic sine of a
COSH(A)	hyperbolic cosine of a
ARCOS(C)	arc cosine of c (i.e., angle for which c is cosine)
ARSIN(S)	arc sine of s
ATAN2(T1,T2)	arc tangent of t_1/t_2

As mentioned before, all arguments are in radians for the first five of these functions. For the last three, however, the returned result, rather than the argument, is in radians.

Manipulative Routines

We listed earlier ABS for absolute value. As in the case of the other functions we have listed, the argument must be in real mode. However, we now add

IABS(J)   absolute value, integer argument

Two functions are designed to obtain the value of an argument, with *sign* matching that of a *second* argument. Thus

SIGN(A,B)   returns the value A, with the same sign as B

For integers,

ISIGN(K,L)   returns the value K, with the same sign as L

For example, our rounding statement

$$X = X + .005 * (X/ABS(X))$$

could be written,

$$X = X + SIGN(.005,X)$$

Another function having to do with sign of results performs a subtraction if the first argument is larger than the second, but produces *zero* if it is smaller. Thus

DIM(C,D)   If c > d, returns the value (c − d)
              If c ≤ d, returns 0

For $C = 7.0$, $D = 3.0$, the function produces $A = 4.0$. But for $C = 3.0$, $D = 7.0$, the value returned is zero. The equivalent for integer arguments is

IDIM(L,M)

Four separate functions deal with selection of the largest of a number of arguments. (They differ from our "BIG" function subprogram in that they require as arguments the individual variables that are to be compared.) Any number of arguments may appear.

AMAX1(W,X,Y,Z ...)   returns the largest of the values mentioned; note that the arguments are in *real* mode, and so is the returned value

AMAX0(K,L,M,N, ...)   is used to select the largest of a set of *integer* arguments—but the value returned is in *real* mode

MAX1(W,X,Y,Z, ...)   selects the largest of a set of *real* arguments, but returns a value in *integer* mode

and finally,

MAX0(K,L,M,N, ...)   selects the largest of a set of *integer* arguments and returns that value in *integer* mode

Four functions are available to do the opposite—that is, to select the *smallest* of the arguments. The meanings parallel those of the "MAX" routines, substituting "MIN":

AMIN1	real arguments, real value returned
AMIN0	integer arguments, real value returned
MIN1	real arguments, integer value returned
MIN0	integer arguments, integer value returned

A usage example may illustrate some of these distinctions. Let the "mid-range" be defined as

$$\frac{\text{highest value} - \text{lowest value}}{2}$$

Then for real arguments, the following statements are valid:

(1)   RANGM = (AMAX1(A,B,C) − AMIN1(A,B,C))/2.0

This statement both uses and produces real values, so that RANGM may have decimal content. But

(2)   RANGM = (MAX1(A,B,C) − MIN1(A,B,C))/2

produces integer subtraction and division of truncated values on the right side, resulting in RANGM without decimal content (and does not work correctly if A, B, and C are very large or very small real values!). For integer arguments, the legal expressions would be:

(1)   RANGM = (AMAX0(I,J,K) − AMIN0(I,J,K))/2.0

or

(2)   RANGM = (MAX0(I,J,K) − MIN0(I,J,K))/2

As another example, the job of our RATIO subprogram could be reduced to a single statement, by use of the appropriate FORTRAN-supplied functions:

```
      --------------
      IF (X − Y) 100, 100, 101
  100 RATIO = X/Y
      --------------          is replaced by
  101 RATIO = Y/X
      --------------
                              RATIO = AMIN1(X,Y)/AMAX1(X,Y)
```

TABLE 19

FORTRAN-Supplied Functions

	TAN	COTAN	SINH COSH	TANH	ARCOS	ARSIN	ATAN2	IABS	SIGN	ISIGN	DIM
1[a]				√				√	√	√	
2				√				√	√	√	
3				√				√	√	√	√
4				√			√	√	√	ASIGN	√
5	√	√	√	√	√	√	√	√	√	√	√
6				√			√	√	√	√	√
7									SIGNF		
8								XABSF	SIGNF		
9	TANF			TANHF	ACOSF	ASINF		XABSF	SIGNF	XSIGNF	DIMF
10				√				√	√	√	
11								√	√	√	
12								√	√	√	√
13	√	COTF		√	ACOS	ASIN	√	√	√	√	√
14	√			√	ACOS	ASIN	√	√	√	√	√
15	√			√	ACOS	ASIN	√	√	√	√	√
16	TANF			TANHF				XABSF	SIGNF	XSIGNF	DIMF
17						ASIN		XABS	√	XSIGN	√
18				√				√	√	√	
19											
20											
21				√			√	√	√	√	√
22			√	√	ACOS	ASIN	√	√	√	√	√
23				√			√	√	√	√	√
24				√			√	√	√	√	√
25								√			
26				√			√	√	√	√	√
27								XABSF	SIGNF	XSIGNF	DIMF
28				√				√	√	√	
29				√			√	√	√	√	√
30				√				√	√	√	√
31								XABSF	SIGNF	XSIGNF	DIMF
32	TANF	COTF			ACOSF	ASINF		XABSF	SIGNF	XSIGNF	
33				√			√	√	√	√	√
34				√			√	√	√	√	√
35			SINHG COSHF	TANHF				XABSF	SIGNF	XSIGNF	DIMF
36								XABSF	√	√	

[a] Compiler number.
[b] Without the terminal F character.
[c] And HFIX.

IDIM	AMAX1 AMAX0 MAX1 MAX0	AMIN1 AMIN0 MIN1 MIN0	MAX1F MAX0F XMAX1F XMAX0F	MIN1F MIN0F XMIN1F XMIN0F	AINT	INT	IFIX	FLOAT	AMOD	MOD
							√	√		
	√	√			√	√	√	√	√	√
√	√	√			√	√	√	√	√	√
	AMAX1 AMAX0	MIN1 MIN0								
√	√	√			√	√	√	√	√	√
√	√	√			√	√		√	√	√
							FIX			
XDIMF			√	√	INTF	XINTF	XFIXF	FLOATF	MODF	XMODF
							√	√		
							√	√		
√					√	√	√	√	√	√
√	√	√			√	√	√	√	√	√
√	√	√			√	√	√	√	√	√
√	√	√			√	√	√	√	√	√
XDIMF			√	√	INTF	XINTF			MODF	XMODF
XDIM			√ [b]	√ [b]	INT	XINT	XFIX	√	√	XMOD
							√	√		
	AMAXI MAXI	AMINI MINI								
√					√	√	√	√	√	√
√	√	√			√	√	√	√	√	√
√	√	√			√	√	√	√	√	√
√	√	√			√	√	√	√	√	√
√	√	√			√	√	√	√	√	√
XDIMF			√	√	INTF	XINTF	XFIXF	FLOATF	MODF	XMODF
							√	√		
√	√	√			√	√	√ [c]	√	√	√
√	√	√			√	√	√	√	√	√
XDIMF			√	√	XINTF	XINTF	XFIXF	FLOATF	MODF	XMODF
			√	√	INTF	XINTF	XFIXF	FLOATF	MODF	XMODF
√	√	√			√	√	√	√	√	√
√	√	√			√	√	√	√	√	√
XDIMF			√	√	INTF	XINTF	XFIXF	FLOATF	MODF	XMODF
	√	√	√	√	√	√	√	√	√	√

TABLE 19 (*continued*)

	TAN	COTAN	SINH COSH	TANH	ARCOS	ARSIN	ATAN2	IABS	SIGN	ISIGN	DIM
37				√			√	√	√	√	√
38				√			√	√	√	√	√
39				√			√	√	√	√	√
40				√				√	√	√	√
41				√			√	√	√	√	√
42	√	√	√	√	√	√	√	√	√	√	√
43	√	√	√	√	√	ARCSIN	√	√	√	√	√
44				√				√	√	√	
45								XABSF			
46								XABSF	SIGNF	XSIGNF	DIMF
47								√	√	√	√
48											
49				√				√	√	√	
50								√	√	√	
51				√	√	√	√	√	√	√	√
52	√	√	√	√	√	√	√	√	√	√	√
53				TANHF		ASINF		XABSF	SIGNF	XSIGNF	DIMF
54								√	√	√	√
55	√	√	√	√	√	√	√	√	√	√	√
56	√	COT	√	√	ACOS	ASIN	√	√	√	√	√
57	TANF			TANHF	ACOSF	ASINF		IABSF	SIGNF	ISIGNF	DIMF
58	TANF			TANHF	ACOSF	ASINF		IABSF	SIGNF	ISIGNF	DIMF
59		[Not stated]									
60				√			√	√	√	√	√
61				√			√	√	√	√	√
62	TANF										
63	√	√	√	√	√	√	√	√	√	√	√
64				√			√	√	√	√	√
65				TANHF				XABSF	SIGNF	XSIGNF	DIMF
66				√			√	√	√	√	√
67				√				√	√	√	
68[d]			√	√			√	√	√	√	√
69[d]	√		√	√	ACOS	ASIN	√	√	√	√	√
70				√			√	√	√	√	√
71				√			√	√	√	√	√
72				√			√	√	√	√	√
73				√		ASIN	√	√	√	√	√
74	√	√			ACOS	ASIN	√	√	√	√	√
75	√		√	√	ACOS	ASIN	√	√	√	√	√
76	√		√	√	ACOS	ASIN	√	√	√	√	√
77	√		√	√	ACOS	ASIN	√	√	√	√	√
78	√		√	√	ACOS	ASIN		√	√	√	√
79				√			√	√	√	√	√

[d] Also accepts some FORTRAN II function titles.

IDIM	AMAX1 AMAX0 MAX1 MAX0	AMIN1 AMIN0 MIN1 MIN0	MAX1F MAX0F XMAX1F XMAX0F	MIN1F MIN0F XMIN1F XMIN0F	AINT	INT	IFIX	FLOAT	AMOD	MOD
√	√	√			√	√	√	√	√	√
√	√	√			√	√	√	√	√	√
√	√	√			√	√	√	√	√	√
√	√	√			√	√	√	√	√	√
√	√	√			√	√	√	√	√	√
√	√	√			√	√	√ (c)	√	√	√
√	√	√			√	√	√ (c)	√	√	√
							√ XFIXF	√ FLOATF		
XDIMF			√	√	INTF	XINTF	XFIXF	FLOATF	MODF	XMODF
√	√	√			√	√	√	√	√	√
	√	√					√	√		
√	√	√			√	√	√	√	√	√
√					√	√	√	√	√	√
√	√	√			√	√	√	√	√	√
XDIMF			√	√	INTF	XINTF	XFIXF	FLOATF	MODF	XMODF
√	√	√			√	√	√	√	√	√
√	√	√			√	√	√	√	√	√
√	√	√			√	√	√	√	√	√
IDIMF	AMAXF MAXF	AMINF MINF			AINTF	INTF	IFIXF	FLOATF	AMODF	MODF
IDIMF	AMAXF MAXF	AMINF MINF			AINTF	INT	IFIXF	FLOATF	AMODF	MODF
√	√	√			√	√	√	√	√	√
√	√	√			√ INTF	√	√ FIXF	√ FLOATF	√	√
√	√	√			√	√	√	√	√	√
√	√	√			√	√	√	√	√	√
XDIMF					INTF	XINTF	XFIXF	FLOATF	MODF	XMODF
√	√	√			√	√	√	√	√	√
							√	√		
√	√	√			√	√	√	√	√	√
√	√	√			√	√	√	√	√	√
√	√	√			√	√	√	√	√	√
√	√	√			√	√	√	√	√	√
√	√	√			√	√	√	√	√	√
√	√	√			√	√	√	√	√	√
√	√	√			√	√	√	√	√	√
√	√	√			√	√	√	√	√	√
√	√	√			√	√	√	√	√	√
√	√	√			√	√	√	√	√	√

Direct truncation of a real value, which eliminates the decimal portion of the number (without rounding), is accomplished by

$$AINT(X)$$

For example, if X = 648258.85, then

$$Y = AINT(X) \quad \text{produces} \quad Y = 648258.0$$

Note that this method truncates numbers that may be too large for a truncation method described in Chapter 5, using conversion from real to integer mode and back again. If the real argument is small enough, however, a truncation providing an *integer* result is accomplished in one step by

$$INT(X)$$

Thus the following statement is valid:

$$K = INT(X) + J \qquad \text{For X} = 648258.85, \text{ and J} = 6,$$
$$\text{the result is } 648264$$

For compilers permitting *mixed expressions* (see Table 10),

$$K = X + J$$

produces the same result. The method used, however, is

$$K = X + FLOAT(J)$$

The FLOAT function converts an integer argument to real mode. Conversion in the other direction, from real to integer, is accomplished by IFIX. Thus

$$K = IFIX(X) + J$$

produces all the arithmetic in integer mode, once again.

Finally, a function is available that produces the "remainder" from any division (first argument divided by the second). For example,

$$R = AMOD(19.0, 4.0)$$

produces R = 3.0 (since the division would produce $4\tfrac{3}{4}$). The equivalent for integer arguments is

$$MOD(19,4)$$

Table 19 shows the availability of these functions in various FORTRAN compilers. (Tables 5 and 19 do not constitute a complete list of available compiler-supplied functions. Those dealing with *complex* and *double precision* variables are listed in Chapter 10, Tables 21 and 22.)

For Review

Examples

calling statement	A = SQRT(B)
statement function	POLYN (A,B,C) = A*X**2+B*X+C
dummy argument	A,B,C
function subprogram	FUNCTION POLYN(A,B,C)
main program	
RETURN statement	RETURN
adjustable DIMENSION	DIMENSION X(K,L)
subroutine subprogram	SUBROUTINE CORR(X,Y,N,A,B,R)
CALL statement	CALL CORR(B,C,K,ADD,XMULT,COEFF)
COMMON statement	COMMON A,B,C
labeled COMMON	COMMON /ONE/A,B,C/TWO/X,Y
EXTERNAL statement	EXTERNAL SIN, COS
ENTRY statement	ENTRY GEOM(N)

EXERCISES

85. The central part of a program says,

```
K = 3
KSEC = NSEC(K, 7*K, 14)
```

Write a statement function that precedes this segment, to return the number of seconds in a time interval stated in the arguments as hours, minutes, and seconds. Add an output statement for KSEC and complete the program for testing.

86. Rewrite your statement function in Exercise 85 as a complete function subprogram; test it by using the original calling program (from which the statement function must be removed).

87. Write a subprogram that converts a time interval of NSEC seconds into the equivalent number of *hours*, *minutes*, and *seconds*. Test it with a calling program that passes 12,074 seconds as the actual argument.

88. Forsyth's approximation for n! is

$$n! = \sqrt{2\pi} \left\{ \frac{\sqrt{n^2 + n + \frac{1}{6}}}{e} \right\}^{n + 1/2}$$

Write a program in which this method appears as a statement function. The program should then compute (a) by actual multiplication, (b) by this method, 10!, 20!, and 30! Output should be in exponential notation, organized to show three lines, each comparing results (a) and (b).

89. Write a function subprogram MIN(I, J, K) that returns the value of the smallest of the three integers I, J, K. Write a calling program that tests the function by using the statement

$$M = MIN(-1,0,2) + MIN(0,-1,2) + MIN(2,0,-1) + MIN(-1,0,-1)$$

90. Write a function subprogram INTCIR(X1, Y1, R1, X2, Y2, R2) that, given two circles—one of radius R1, center at (X1, Y1), the other of radius R2, center at (X2, Y2)—returns a value

       2 if the circles intersect at two points
       1 if the circles are tangent to one another
       0 if they have no points in common
      −1 if they intersect at an infinite number of points

Write a calling program that will read four data sets, call the function four times, and output the four returned values. Use as data

3.	0.	1.	3.	0.	1.
−1.	0.	1.	3.	0.	2.
0.	0.	1.	3.	0.	2.
1.	0.	1.	3.	0.	2.

91. Write a function subprogram that will return the smallest value in any argument array (single dimension). Then call it in a program that computes the arithmetic mean of the smallest items on each of the 20 data cards (i.e., the function will be called 20 times, on each occasion for five items).

92. Write a function subprogram that returns the arithmetic mean of the *diagonal* elements (1, 1), (2, 2), etc., of any *square* array (use adjustable dimensions, if your compiler permits; otherwise, write the subprogram for a maximum of 20 × 20). Call the subprogram with a program that treats the first 25 data items as a 5 × 5 array and prints the returned result.

93. Write a subroutine subprogram that will convert *radians* to degrees, minutes, and seconds. Make use of the relationships:

       1 degree = .0174532925 radians
       1 minute = .0002908882 radians
       1 second = .0000048481 radians

Write a calling program that calls the subprogram for 1, 3, 5, 7, and 9 radians and outputs the results.

94. Write a subprogram that will return the *harmonic mean* of n elements of the X array, when called by the statement

CALL HARMF(X,N,HMEAN)

The harmonic mean is defined as the reciprocal of the mean reciprocal:

$$H = \frac{n}{\sum \frac{1}{X}}$$

Write a calling program that reads ten array elements, calls the subprogram, and outputs the returned result.

95. Rewrite the *sorting* program in Exercise 66 as the subroutine subprogram

SUBROUTINE ORDER(A,L,N).

Test the subprogram with a calling program that reads three sets of ten items each and calls the subprogram (which performs the output activities) for each set.

96. Write a subroutine subprogram to obtain (and output) the least-squares linear regression equation and the correlation coefficient, for n values of X and Y. (This is a minor modification of Exercise 54.) Let n be an argument and let X and Y values be stored in COMMON. Then write a calling program that first obtains a, b, and r for actual X and Y values and then for natural *logarithms* of the X and Y values. (Test on the first six data items treated as X values and the next six as Y values.)

97. Adjust the subprogram in Exercise 96 by placing a and b in COMMON. Then write a calling program that produces a *semilogarithmic trend equation* for the first ten data items, treated as Y values. That is, the logarithms of these (annual values) will be considered a linear function of *time* (X), which will be coded as *zero* through *nine*. The calling program must generate X values 0 through 9. After the subprogram has been called, let the calling program output "projections" of Y_c for years 10, 11, 12, and 13 (i.e., the 11th through 14th actual years).

98. Write a function subprogram called SUMSQ that will return the *sum of the squares* of the ith through jth elements of the X array (specifying one real and two integer arguments). That is, the returned result is

$$\sum X^2$$

Also write one called SQSUM that will return the *squared sum* of the ith through jth elements of the X array; that is, the returned result is

$$(\sum X)^2$$

Test both functions with a calling program using the 11th to 20th data items (having read the entire data deck as a one-dimension array). Then put both aside for later use (Chapter 12).

10 • OTHER VARIABLE TYPES

We have discussed two major types of variables: real ("floating point") and integer ("fixed point"). Three other types are available in some compilers: *Double Precision, Complex,* and *Logical.* There is no implicit specification system[1] for any of these types (such as the first-character distinction between real and integer variables). Therefore the programmer must declare the special status by using explicit type specification statements:

```
DOUBLE PRECISION X,Y,B(12)
COMPLEX GAUGE, CROSS(10)
LOGICAL MAN, BOY, PARENT(2)
```

When a *subscripted* variable is to be typed by one of these statements, dimension information should appear within the statement and should not then be repeated in subsequent specification statements.

Double Precision

Double precision variables are effectively in real mode, but are stored in "longer" locations that permit representation of numbers with greater *precision* (approximately twice as many significant digits) than the ordinary (single precision) real variable. As Table 6 (Chapter 3) indicated, single precision real constants have typically between 7 and 11 significant digits. Table 20 shows that many systems permit from 14 to 25 digits in double precision constants. The table also indicates availability of the DOUBLE PRECISION explicit type specification, which reserves the extra-length storage locations. In some systems, the choice of double precision must be made for all real variables at once, by use of a *control card* rather than a specification statement. This method will receive some discussion in Chapter 12.

---

[1] An exception is arranged by the IMPLICIT statement, discussed in Chapter 11.

TABLE 20

Double Precision

| | Declaration | | | Precision | D Notation | | | |
| | Explicit Type Specification | Control Card | Not Available | Number of Digits | Mandatory | | Optional | Not Used |
					All	Less Than N Digits		
1[a]			✓					
2			✓					
3	✓			2 × number specified for REAL (by control card)	✓			
4			✓					
5	✓			23	✓			
6	✓			16		8		
7			✓					
8			✓					
9	✓ Type double			25	✓			
10			✓					
11			✓					
12			✓					
13	✓			25	✓			
14	✓			29	✓			
15	✓			29	✓			
16		✓[b]		12				✓
17		✓[b]		12				✓
18			✓					
19			✓					
20			✓					
21	✓			9	✓			
22	✓			16	✓			
23	✓			Not stated			✓	
24	✓			Not stated			✓	
25			✓					
26			✓					
27			✓					

[a] Compiler number.

[b] Double unless controlled.

TABLE 20 (*continued*)

| | Declaration | | | Precision Number of Digits | D Notation | | | |
| | Explicit Type Specification | Control Card | Not Available | | Mandatory | | Optional | Not Used |
					All	Less Than N Digits		
28			√					
29	√			16			√	
30			√					
31			√					
32			√					
33			√					
34	√			18			√	
35			√					
36			√					
37		√		2–20				√
38	√			13 predecimal 7 postdecimal	√			
39	√			Not stated	√			
40	√			16		8		
41	√			16		8		
42	√			16		8		
43	√			16		8		
44		√		10				√
45		√		20 maximum				√
46		√		45 maximum				√
47		√		20 maximum				√
48			√					
49		√		10				√
50		√		18 maximum				√
51			√					
52	√			17			√	
53			√					
54			√					
55	√			16		10		
56	√			20	√			
57			√					

TABLE 20 (*continued*)

	Declaration			Precision Number of Digits	D Notation Mandatory		Optional	Not Used
	Explicit Type Specification	Control Card	Not Available		All	Less Than N Digits		
58			√					
59			√					
60	√			21			√	
61	√			21	√			
62			√					
63	√			19		14		
64	√			16			√	
65			√					
66			√					
67			√					
68	√			18	√			
69	√	or √		15	√			
70	√			15	√			
71	√			11	√			
72	√			18	√			
73	√			11			√	
74	√			17	√			
75	√			14		6		
76	√			17	√			
77	√			18	√			
78			√					
79	√			No ruling	√			

The usefulness of the double precision arrangement to the programmer arises in several situations. First, some problems require accuracy to a greater number of digits than single precision provides. The use of π as a constant might be restricted to

$$PI = 3.1415927$$

in single precision. But

```
DOUBLE PRECISION PI, ANS
PI = 3.1415926535897932
```

may be useful for a problem in which a highly precise answer is needed.

A second advantage of double precision accrues to programmers using what we have earlier called "straight binary" computers. In such systems the postdecimal portions of numbers are frequently stored in binary form, separately from the predecimal portions. This results in approximate representation— "rounding error"—of decimals that do not correspond exactly to sums of available negative powers of the base 2. Since double precision increases the range of these negative powers, it results in closer approximations (less "rounding error"—in effect, rounding error is pushed further to the right of the number).

A third advantage of double precision is observable in Table 11 (Chapter 6): the length of the *alphameric string* that may be stored as a single variable is frequently greater, for double precision variables.

Although we have represented the double precision constant in ordinary decimal notation in the example above, many systems require a different form, particularly for smaller double precision constants. The form is actually exponential notation written with "D" rather than "E." For example,

$$3.1415926535897932D+00$$
$$\text{or}\quad 1.5D-10$$
$$\text{or}\quad 3.75D+13$$

Table 20 indicates the applicable rules in various systems.

The FORMAT description used for input and output of double precision values depends on whether the values are handled with or without the "D" notation. The usual F specification may be used for input where the system permits ordinary decimal notation for double precision constants, and for output when the programmer does not want the "D" notation to appear.

```
      --------------------
          DOUBLE PRECISION PI
   30     FORMAT (F19.16)
   31     FORMAT (F8.5)
          READ (2,30) PI
          WRITE (2,30) PI
          WRITE (2,31) PI

      --------------------
```

This segment reads an input value punched in decimal notation and produces as output:

$$\text{b}3.1415926535897932$$
$$\text{b}3.14159$$

When D notation is used, the general form is Dw.d; our FORMAT specifications become

      30   FORMAT (D23.16)

      31   FORMAT (D12.5)

producing

    b3.1415926535897932D+00   (which also appears on the input record)

    b3.14159D+00

As with E notation, a minimum difference of 6 is required between w and d, to allow room for decimal point, sign, and four characters of D notation.

The mixture of single and double precision variables on the right side of arithmetic expressions *is* permitted. The result is temporary conversion of the single precision value to double precision form for the computation; therefore such arithmetic is carried on in double precision form, even though some of the values are not declared double precision by the programmer. This conversion feature, permitting "mixed" expressions, was mentioned in Chapter 5 with respect to conversion of integer values to real mode. Systems that permit full use of mixed expressions follow a hierarchy rule as follows:

      (high)   Complex

                   Double Precision

                   Real

      (low)   Integer

The "low" order modes are converted to higher order when used in mixed expressions. The "conversion" does not change the stored value. Note that *logical* values cannot usually appear in mixed expressions.

As usually, the variable on the *left* of the equal-sign in an arithmetic statement may be in any mode, since conversion of the right-hand result to the left-hand mode is automatically arranged. (Hierarchy rules do not apply.) Therefore, in

DOUBLE PRECISION PI, V, V1

V = PI/V1

V1 = PI/2.0

X = PI/2.0

K = PI/2.0

----

all arithmetic statements are valid. The first contains only double precision variables. The second is evaluated in double precision by temporary conversion of the single precision constant for the arithmetic, and the result is stored in the double precision location V1. In the third, the same result is truncated to single precision, for storage in the X location. The result of the fourth expression is stored in the integer location K, as the predecimal portion of the double precision arithmetic. (For PI = 3.1415926535897932, K = 1.)

Double Precision Functions

Many of the FORTRAN-supplied functions are duplicated for the special case of double precision arguments (and return double precision results). A "D" appears in front of the usual function title. These are:

DLOG	logarithm (base e)
DLOG10	logarithm (base 10)
DEXP	antilogarithm (base e)
DSQRT	square root
DSIN	sine
DCOS	cosine

TABLE 21

FORTRAN-Supplied Double Precision Functions

	No Double Precision	By Control Card—Real Functions Apply	DLOG	DLOG10	DSQRT DEXP	DSIN DCOS	DATAN	DATAN2	DTAN
1[a]	√								
2	√								
3			√	√	√	√	√	√	
4	√								
5			√	√	√	√	√	√	
6			√	√	√	√	√	√	
7	√								
8	√								
9			√		√	√	√		
10	√								
11	√								
12	√								

[a] Compiler number.

DATAN		arctangent							

DATAN · · · arctangent
DATAN2 · · · arctangent of t_1/t_2
DTANH · · · hyperbolic tangent

DABS · · · absolute value
DMAX1 · · · largest of arguments
DMIN1 · · · smallest of arguments
DSIGN · · · a_1 gets sign of a_2
DFLOAT · · · convert from integer to double precision form
DINT · · · truncate the double precision argument (equivalent to AINT)
IDINT · · · convert from double precision to integer form (equivalent to INT)
DREAL · · · extract real portion of complex double precision argument [2]
DIMAG · · · extract imaginary portion of complex double precision argument [2]

[2] See next section and Table 24.

DTANH	DABS	DMAX1 DMIN1	DSIGN DMOD	DFLOAT	IDINT	DINT	SNGL DBLE	DREAL DIMAG
	√	√	√		√		√	
	√	√	√		√		√	
	√	√	√		√		√	

TABLE 21 (*continued*)

	No Double Precision	By Control Card—Real Functions Apply	DLOG	DLOG10	DSQRT DEXP	DSIN DCOS	DATAN	DATAN2	DTAN
13			√	√	√	√	√	√	
14			√	√	√	√	√	√	
15			√	√	√	√	√	√	
16		√							
17		√							
18	√								
19	√								
20	√								
21			√	√	√	√	√	√	
22			√	√	√	√	√	√	
23			√	√	√	√	√	√	
24			√	√	√	√	√	√	
25	√								
26	√								
27	√								
28	√								
29			√	√	√	√	√	√	
30	√								
31	√								
32	√								
33	√								
34			√	√	√	√	√	√	
35	√								
36	√								
37		√							
38			√	√	√	√	DTAN	DTAN2	
39			√	√	√	√	√	√	
40			√	√	√	√	√		
41			√	√	√	√	√	√	
42			√	√	√	√	√	√	√
43			√	√	√	√	√	√	√
44		√							
45		√							

DTANH	DABS	DMAX1 DMIN1	DSIGN DMOD	DFLOAT	IDINT	DINT	SNGL DBLE	DREAL DIMAG
	√	√	√		√		√	
	√	√	√		√		√	
	√	√	√		√		√	
		DMAXI DMINI						
	√		√		√		√	
	√		√		√		√	
	√	√	√		√		√	
	√	√	√		√		√	
	√	√	√	√	√	√	√	√
	√	√	√		√		√	
		DMAXI DMIN						
	√		√		√		√	
	√	√	√		√		√	
√	√	√	√	√	√		√	
√	√	√	√	√	√		√	
√	√	√	√	√	√		√	
√	√	√	√	√	√		√	

TABLE 21 (*continued*)

	No Double Precision	By Control Card—Real Functions Apply	DLOG	DLOG10	DSQRT DEXP	DSIN DCOS	DATAN	DATAN2	DTAN
46		√							
47		√							
48	√								
49		√							
50		√							
51	√								
52			√	√	√	√	√	√	
53	√								
54	√								
55			√	√	√	√	√	√	
56			√	√	√	√	√	√	
57	√								
58	√								
59	√								
60			√	√	√	√	√	√	
61			√	√	√	√	√	√	
62	√								
63			√	√	√	√		DTAN2	
64			√	√	√	√	√	√	
65	√								
66	√								
67	√								
68			√	√	√	√	√	√	
69			√	√	√	√	√	√	
70			√	√	√	√	√	√	
71			√	√	√	√	DTAN	√	
72			√	√	√	√	DTAN	√	
73			√	√	√	√	√	√	
74			√	√	√	√	√	√	√
75			BLOG	√	√	√	√	√	√
76			√	√	√	√	√	√	√
77			√	√	√	√	√	√	√
78	√								
79			√	√	√	√	√	√	

DTANH	DABS	DMAX1 DMIN1	DSIGN DMOD	DFLOAT	IDINT	DINT	SNGL DBLE	DREAL DIMAG
	√	√	√		√		√	
	√	√	√		√		√	
	√	√	√		√		√	
	√	√	√		√		√	
	√	√	√		√	√	√	
	√	√	√		√		√	
	√	√	√	√	√	√	√	√
	√	√	√		√	√	√	
√	√	√	√	√	√	√	√	
√	√	√	√	√	√		√ SNGLE	
	√	√	√		√		DBLE	
							SNGLE	
	√	√	√		√		DBLE	
	√	√	√		√		√	
	√	√	√	√	√		√	
	√	√	√		√		√	
√	√	√	√			√	√	
√	√	√	√		√	√	√	
	√	√	√		√		√	

In addition, two new functions deal with double precision values. They are both concerned with conversion between single and double precision form.

(1)
$$\begin{array}{c} \text{DOUBLE PRECISION V} \\ \hline \text{A = X + SNGL(V)} \end{array}$$

This calls for conversion of V to single precision form for the computation. The opposite is achieved by

(2)   V = DBLE(X) + V

which converts X to double precision form (somewhat redundantly, since most systems make this conversion automatically, as stated earlier).

Table 21 shows the availability of double precision functions in various FORTRAN compilers.

Complex Variables

The information in this section is of little value to those of us (I must include myself) who do not use *complex quantities* in the usual course of events. If the value

$$5.0 + 2.0i$$

where $i = \sqrt{-1}$ has no meaning to you, you will not miss anything by skipping to the section on Logical variables.

Those who remain will recognize that $i = \sqrt{-1}$ (an imaginary number) and that the value above would be obtained as one of the roots of[3]

$$3X^2 - 30X + 87 = 0$$

Complex numbers are always of the general form

$$a + bi$$
$$c + di$$

They may be handled in computation, but the rules are highly specialized. You may remember that the product of the two values above is

$$(ac - bd) + (ad + bc)i$$

---

[3] Using the quadratic solution formula

$$\frac{-b \pm \sqrt{b^2 - 4ac}}{2a} = \frac{30 \pm \sqrt{900 - 1044}}{6} = \frac{30 \pm \sqrt{-144}}{6} = \frac{30 \pm 12\sqrt{-1}}{6} = 5 \pm 2i$$

and their quotient is

$$\frac{ac + bd}{c^2 + d^2} + \frac{bc - ad}{c^2 + d^2} \, i$$

FORTRAN provides automatic implementation of such computation formulas, as well as some more complicated ones, when the programmer declares any variable to be in complex form.

```
      COMPLEX X,Y,PROD,QUOT,SUM,SUBTR,POWER
10    FORMAT (E16.8, F10.1, 2F12.4)
      READ (2,10) X,Y
      PROD = X * Y
      QUOT = X/Y
      SUM = X + Y
      SUBTR = X − Y
      POWER = X**5
```

Each of the usual arithmetic operations is available.[4] Note that the FORMAT statement may use ordinary F or E notation as required, but must provide *two* specifications for each complex value.

Complex constants are written with parentheses enclosing the two components (both in real mode), which are separated by a comma. Thus the sample segment might continue:

```
      X = X + (6.0,3.25)
      Y = Y/X * (17.1,4.0)
      PROD = X * Y * (0.0,4.5)
```

In the last instance, the constant value is 4.5i; the zero must be mentioned, as illustrated.

Complex and simple real values may be mixed in arithmetic expressions, just as they are in mathematical usage. The result is always a complex value. For example,

```
      COMPLEX C

      C = C + X
```

In this case X is used as a complex value, with zero for its imaginary part.

---

[4] For the ** operator, the exponent must be in integer mode.

Complex Functions

Three kinds of specialized FORTRAN-supplied functions apply to complex values.

First, many of the usual functions are duplicated for complex arguments (and return a complex result); they are designated by "C" in front of the usual symbol:

CLOG	logarithm (base e)
CLOG10	logarithm (base 10)
CEXP	antilogarithm (base e)
CSQRT	square root
CSIN	sine
CCOS	cosine
CABS	absolute value

Second, certain functions deal with complex arguments in *double precision* form:

CDLOG	logarithm (base e)
CDLG10	logarithm (base 10)
CDEXP	antilogarithm (base e)
CDSQRT	square root
CDSIN	sine
CDCOS	cosine
CDABS	absolute value
CSNGL	convert to single precision form
CDBLE	convert to double precision form

Third, four new functions apply only to manipulation of complex values:

(1)
$$\begin{array}{c} \text{COMPLEX X} \\ \hline \text{A = REAL(X) + B} \end{array}$$

The REAL function returns the first (real)[5] portion of the complex value.

(2)   A = AIMAG(X) + B

The AIMAG function returns the second (imaginary) portion of the complex value (using it as a real number, disregarding i).

----

[5] "Real" is here used in the mathematical, not the programming, sense.

TABLE 22

FORTRAN-Supplied Complex Functions

	No Complex	CLOG	CLOG10	CSQRT CEXP	CSIN CCOS	CABS	REAL AIMAG	CMPLX CONJG	CDLOG	CDLG10	CDSQRT CDEXP	CDSIN CDCOS	CDABS	CSNGL CDBLE	DCMPLX DCONJG
1[a]	✓														
2	✓														
3	✓														
4		✓													
5		✓		✓	✓	✓	✓	✓							
6		✓		✓	✓	✓	✓	✓							
7	✓														
8	✓														
9					[No complex functions]										
10	✓														
11	✓														
12	✓														
13		✓		✓	✓	✓	✓	✓							
14		✓		✓	✓	✓	✓	✓							
15		✓		✓	✓	✓	✓	✓							
16	✓														
17	✓														
18	✓														
19	✓														
20	✓														
21	✓														
22		✓		✓	✓	✓	✓	✓							
23		✓		✓	✓	✓	✓	✓							
24		✓		✓	✓	✓	✓	✓							
25	✓														
26	✓														
27	✓														

[a] Compiler number.

TABLE 22 (*continued*)

No.	No Complex	CLOG / CLOG10	CSQRT / CEXP	CSIN / CCOS	CABS	REAL / AIMAG	CMPLX / CONJG	CDLOG	CDLG10	CDSQRT / CDEXP	CDSIN / CDCOS	CDABS	CSNGL / CDBLE	DCMPLX / DCONJG
28	✓													
29	✓	✓		✓	✓	✓	✓	✓			✓	✓	✓	✓
30	✓		✓	✓	✓	✓	✓			✓	✓	✓	✓	✓
31	✓													
32	✓													
33	✓													
34	✓	✓	✓	✓	✓	✓	✓							
35	✓													
36	✓													
37	✓	✓												
38			✓	✓	✓	✓	✓							
39			✓	✓	✓	✓	✓							
40	✓	✓												
41	✓									✓	✓			
42			✓	✓	✓	✓	✓			✓	✓	✓		✓
43	✓	✓	✓	✓	✓	✓	✓	✓		✓	✓	✓		✓
44	✓													
45	✓													
46	✓													
47	✓													
48	✓													
49	✓													
50	✓													
51	✓													

TABLE 22 (*continued*)

	No Complex	CLOG	CLOG10	CSQRT CEXP	CSIN CCOS	CABS	REAL AIMAG	CMPLX CONJG	CDLOG	CDLG10	CDSQRT CDEXP	CDSIN CDCOS	CDABS	CSNGL CDBLE	DCMPLX DCONJG
52		✓		✓	✓	✓	✓	✓							
53	✓														
54	✓														
55		✓		✓	✓	✓	✓								
56		✓		✓	✓	✓	✓	✓							
57	✓							✓							
58	✓														
59	✓														
60		✓		✓	✓	✓	✓	✓							
61		✓		✓	✓	✓	✓	✓							
62	✓				✓		✓	✓							
63		✓		✓	✓		✓	✓							
64		✓		✓	✓	✓	✓	✓	✓		✓	✓	✓		
65	✓										✓	✓	✓	✓	✓
66	✓										✓	✓	✓	✓	✓
67	✓														
68		✓	✓	✓	✓	✓	✓	✓	✓		✓	✓	✓		
69		✓	✓	✓	✓	✓	✓	✓	✓	✓	✓	✓	✓		✓
70	✓	✓		✓	✓	✓	✓	✓	✓		✓	✓	✓		
71	✓	✓		✓	✓	✓	✓	✓			✓	✓	✓		✓
72	✓	✓		✓	✓	✓	✓	✓							
73	✓														
74	✓														
75	✓														
76		✓		✓	✓	✓	✓	✓							
77		✓		✓	✓	✓	✓	✓							
78	✓														
79		✓		✓	✓	✓	✓	✓							

(3)   X = CMPLX(A,B)

The CMPLX function combines any two real arguments into a complex value. The arguments may be real variables, constants, or arithmetic expressions. Thus

COMPLEX V,Y

V = CMPLX(A, B+6.3)
Y = CMPLX(B, 8.0)

are both valid. Note that the last statement is correct form, whereas the expression in parentheses would *not* be recognized as a legal complex *constant*. That is,

Y = (B,8.0)

would not be legal.

The complex *conjugate* of a complex number is defined:

conj (a + bi) = (a − bi)

This is supplied by the fourth new function; for example,

(4)   V = CONJG(V)

Finally, the last two functions named (CMPLX and CONJG) are available for double precision arguments (and return double precision complex values):

V = DCOMPLX(A,B)
V = DCONJG(V)

Table 22 shows the availability situation for the COMPLEX declaration and for each of the FORTRAN-supplied functions applicable to complex values.

Logical Variables

As we have seen, the declaration of variables as Double Precision or Complex does not alter the programmer's usual intention of performing arithmetic computation (and input/output activities) using real numbers. But the declaration of any variable as LOGICAL conveys a rather different purpose. A logical variable has only two possible values: TRUE or FALSE. Logical *constants* are represented as one of these two words, surrounded by decimal points:

> LOGICAL MAN, BOY, CHILD
> MAN = .TRUE.
> BOY = .FALSE.

Obviously, variables such as these cannot be combined either with other logical[6] or with arithmetic variables, in arithmetic. However, their values may be defined (or changed) by *logical expressions*, which may contain to the right of the equal-sign arithmetic variables and/or constants, and the *relational and logical operators* that we listed in Chapter 7. Thus

> MAN = AGE1 .GE. 21.0

If "AGE1," a real variable, is equal to or greater than 21.0, the MAN will be stored as "TRUE." If AGE1 is less than 21.0, MAN will be stored as "FALSE." Suppose that this is followed by the statements

> BOY = AGE2 .LT. 21.0
> IF (MAN .AND. BOY) DIFF = AGE1 − AGE2
> IF (.NOT. (MAN .AND. BOY)) GO TO 1
> BOY = DIFF .GT. AGE1 * .1

We have noted earlier that Logical IF statement could be used with real or integer expressions in the brackets. We now observe that this is the *only* proper form for use with logical variables, that is, the arithmetic IF statement would be inappropriate.[7]

The statement following the parentheses of "IF" will be executed only if the bracketed expression is TRUE. In our sample sequence, DIFF is computed only if AGE1 is equal to or greater than 21.0 *and* AGE2 is less than 21.0. Without using logical variables, the first IF statement might say:

> IF (AGE1 .GE. 21.0 .AND. AGE2 .LT. 21.0) DIFF = AGE1 − AGE2

---

[6] With two exceptions; a simple equality statement and a comparison. Thus MAN = BOY would give MAN the current value (TRUE or FALSE) of BOY.

> IF (MAN − BOY)1, 2, 1

branches to statement 2 only if both variables have the same logical value (i.e., both .TRUE. or both .FALSE.).

[7] With the exception noted in footnote 6.

The second IF statement in the sample segment arranges for a transfer to statement 1 only if DIFF has not been computed. If it has, the logical variable BOY will be changed to FALSE if the age difference is less than (or equal to) 10 per cent of AGE1.

In the second IF statement, the inner parentheses are required, because the order of precedence of the *logical operators* is:

(highest precedence)	.NOT.
	.AND.
(lowest precedence)	.OR.

You should see, therefore, that removal of the inner brackets would change the meaning to "GO TO 1 only if MAN is FALSE and BOY is TRUE." As another illustration,

```
LOGICAL G, H, I, J, K, L
_____
_____
G = H .AND. I .OR. J .AND. .NOT. K .OR. L
```

As written, the statement has implied brackets,

$$G = (H \text{ .AND. } I) \text{ .OR. } (J \text{ .AND. } (\text{.NOT. } K)) \text{ .OR. } L$$

Thus G is TRUE if *either*

	(1) H and I are TRUE
or	(2) J is TRUE and K is FALSE
or	(3) L is TRUE

If actual brackets are added in any other pattern, the meaning changes:

$$G = H \text{ .AND. } (I \text{ .OR. } J) \text{ .AND. } (\text{NOT. } (K \text{ .OR. } L))$$

G is *now* TRUE *only* if

	(1) H is TRUE
and	(2) I or J is TRUE
and	(3) K and L are FALSE.

Input and output of logical variables require a new FORMAT specification, of the general form

Lw

For output, the variable is represented at the *right* of the requested field as simply T or F.[8] Thus

WRITE (2,100) MAN
100   FORMAT (L5)

produces

bbbbT

or

bbbbF

For input, however, the data item must *begin* with T or F, but may contain any other following characters. Thus

READ (2,99) MAN, BOY
99   FORMAT (2L6)

could refer to a data card keypunched,

TbbbbbFbbbbb

or

TRUEbbFALSEb

or

THOMASFRANKb

Only the first letter, however, is available for output purposes.

If you get the feeling that you could invent substitutes for the *logical variable* (e.g., an integer variable that had values "zero" or "one"), you are, of course, perfectly correct. However, there are some problems—indeed, entire subject areas, such as symbolic logic—in which the logical-variable form is clearer and simpler for the programmer. In addition, we may note that "IF" statements with logical variables as arguments generally are executed at greater speed than arithmetic IF statements.

For a sample of a full program that uses logical variables, let us make up and solve the following problem: A program is to read 100 data cards each containing three values (a, b, c), representing lengths of the three sides of various triangles. The program is to determine which are right triangles (condition: the square of one side is equal to the sum of the squares of the other two sides). Output will consist of an identification number (1–100) and T for right triangle, F for other. In addition, a check should be made to ensure that

---

[8] Some compilers produce the full words, TRUE or FALSE.

TABLE 23

Logical Variables—IMPLICIT and EQUIVALENCE Statements

	Logical Variables		IMPLICIT		EQUIVALENCE	
	Yes	No	Yes	No	Yes	No
1[a]		✓		✓	✓	
2	✓			✓	✓	
3	✓			✓	✓	
4	✓			✓	✓	
5	✓			✓	✓	
6	✓			✓	✓	
7		✓		✓		✓
8		✓		✓	✓	
9	✓[b]			✓	✓	
10		✓[c]		✓	✓	
11		✓[c]		✓	✓	
12		✓		✓	✓	
13	✓			✓	✓	
14	✓			✓	✓	
15	✓			✓	✓	
16		✓		✓	✓	
17		✓		✓	✓	
18		✓		✓	✓	
19		✓		✓		✓
20		✓		✓		✓
21	✓			✓	✓	
22	✓		✓		✓	
23	✓			✓	✓	
24	✓			✓	✓	
25		✓		✓	✓	
26	✓			✓	✓	
27	✓			✓	✓	
28		✓		✓	✓	
29	✓		✓		✓	
30		✓		✓	✓	

[a] Compiler number.
[b] Declared by "TYPE LOGICAL."
[c] Compiler does permit Logical IF statement.

TABLE 23 (*continued*)

	Logical Variables		IMPLICIT		EQUIVALENCE	
	Yes	No	Yes	No	Yes	No
31		√		√	√	
32		√		√	√	
33		√		√	√	
34	√			√	√	
35		√		√	√	
36		√		√	√	
37	√			√	√	
38	√			√	√	
39	√			√	√	
40		√		√	√	
41		√		√	√	
42	√		√		√	
43	√		√		√	
44		√		√	√	
45		√		√	√	
46		√		√	√	
47	√			√	√	
48		√		√		√
49		√		√	√	
50		√		√	√	
51		√		√	√	
52	√			√	√	
53		√		√	√	
54		√		√		√
55	√			√	√	
56	√			√	√	
57	√			√	√	
58	√			√	√	
59		√		√	√	
60	√			√	√	
61	√			√	√	
62		√		√		√
63	√			√	√	

TABLE 22 (*continued*)

	Logical Variables		IMPLICIT		EQUIVALENCE	
	Yes	No	Yes	No	Yes	No
64	√		√		√	
65		√		√	√	
66	√			√	√	
67		√		√	√	
68	√			√	√	
69	√		√		√	
70	√		√		√	
71	√			√	√	
72	√			√	√	
73		√		√	√	
74	√			√	√	
75	√			√	√	
76	√			√	√	
77	√		√		√	
78	√			√	√	
79	√			√	√	

no data item is a negative or zero value; if such is encountered, an error message will result (arranged by the programmer).

```
C     RIGHT TRIANGLES
      LOGICAL RIGHT, DATA
      DO 1 K = 1, 100
      READ (2,10) A, B, C
C     CHECK FOR NEGATIVE OR ZERO DATA
      DATA = A .GT. 0. .AND. B .GT. 0. .AND. C .GT. 0.
      IF (.NOT. DATA) GO TO 2
C     CHECK FOR RIGHT-TRIANGLE CONDITION
      A = A**2
      B = B**2
      C = C**2
      RIGHT = A .EQ. B+C .OR. B .EQ. A+C .OR. C .EQ. A+B
1     WRITE (3,11) K, RIGHT
      CALL EXIT
```

```
C    ERROR MESSAGE
2       WRITE (1,12)
        STOP
10      FORMAT (3F10.4)
11      FORMAT (I6,L12)
12      FORMAT (11H DATA ERROR)
        END
```

Table 23 shows availability of logical variables in various FORTRAN compilers. (The table also references two statements discussed at the beginning of Chapter 11.)

For Review	Examples
double precision variable	DOUBLE PRECISION A,B
double precision constant	3.5D+10
D notation	D20.10
mixed expression	
hierarchy rule	complex/double precision/real/integer
double precision function	DSQRT
complex variable	COMPLEX C, D
complex constant	(5.0,2.0)
complex function	CSQRT
logical variable	LOGICAL E,F,G
logical constant	.TRUE. .FALSE.
logical expression	A .GT. B .AND. C
logical notation	L7

EXERCISES

99. Write a program that checks the real *precision* of your computer, with and without the DOUBLE PRECISION declaration, by outputting 1./3., in large Fw.d notation.

100. For two complex numbers (a + bi) and (c + di), the quotient is obtained from

$$\frac{a + bi}{c + di} = \frac{ac + bd}{c^2 + d^2} + \frac{bc - ad}{c^2 + d^2} i$$

Write a subroutine subprogram that returns the result as two real values, operating on four real arguments (which have *not* been declared COMPLEX by explicit type specification).

Then write a calling program that reads the first four data items as actual arguments (i.e., as two successive complex numbers, but without explicit type specification) and calls the function. If your compiler provides COMPLEX variables, arrange for the calling program to check your subprogram answer directly.

101. A *truth table* that frequently appears in logic textbooks shows the logical values (True or False) resulting from various combinations of logical values and logical expressions:

Values of			Expressions			
p and q	p & q	not (p & q)	not p	not q	not p & not q	not p or not q
p true, q true						
p false, q true						
p true, q false						
p false, q false						

Write a program that fills in the 24 values for the table. (You may find it convenient to split it into a subroutine subprogram and a calling program.)

102. A large firm organizes its personnel records as follows (each data card):

Columns	
2–20	employee name
22–25	year of birth
30	1-digit education code
34–35	2-digit occupation code
40	1-digit marital status code
45	1-digit residence area code

Write a program that will read 1300 cards and reprint the names of all employees meeting the following description:

age:	25 to 37, inclusive (assume you are doing this in 1969)
education code:	3
occupation code:	76, or 79, or 84
marital status:	code 0
residence area:	4 or 6

Use Logical variables, if available. Make up a 10-card data deck to test your program.

103. The logical operations of FORTRAN can be used to verify the validity of Boolean algebra identities. Listed below are six important identities often used by logic design engineers to simplify functions. For each case, define the left side of the equation as LS and the right side as RS, using two logical assignment

statements. Then use a set of nested DO loops to assign in turn all possible combinations of True or False values to the variables A, B, and C. (For n variables, there are of course 2^n combinations.)

Arrange the program to print out, with suitable heading, one combination per line, showing the assigned values for all the variables and the truth values for LS and RS. The identity is verified if all LS and RS values agree. (The output form is again a *truth table*; the method of proof is called *complete induction*.)

(1) A or A & B = A

(2) A & (A or B) = A

(3) A or not A & B = A or B

(4) A & (not A or B) = A & B

(5) (A or B) & (not A or C) & (B or C) = (A or B) & (not A or C)

(6) A & B or not A & C or B & C = A & B or not A & C

11 • OTHER NONEXECUTABLE STATEMENTS

As we have seen, nonexecutable statements provide information to the compiler. This information concerns (1) (*Specification* statements) the number and type of locations required for storage of values: DIMENSION, COMMON, REAL, INTEGER, DOUBLE PRECISION, COMPLEX, LOGICAL, EXTERNAL; (2) the form of input and output data: FORMAT, and individual F, E, I, A, H, X, D, and L specifications; and (3) the starting points and titles of subprograms and the ending points of programs and subprograms: FUNCTION, SUBROUTINE, ENTRY, END. In this chapter we consider some additions to each of these groups:

1. IMPLICIT; EQUIVALENCE; DATA.
2. P, G, and T FORMAT specifications; FORMAT specifications treated as data: NAMELIST.
3. BLOCK DATA.

The IMPLICIT Statement

Some compilers permit the programmer to design a partial or complete *implicit specification* system for any individual program. That is, he may establish certain alphabetic characters as specifying, when they appear as initial characters of variable titles, the type of variable as *real*, *integer*, *complex*, or *logical*. This arrangement overrides the usual integer-real predefinitions and makes unnecessary the use of explicit type specification statements. The latter are still permissible, however, and override IMPLICIT for particular variables. Thus

```
IMPLICIT REAL(A,B), INTEGER(C-X), LOGICAL(Y,Z)
REAL TORCH
```

As illustrated, the parentheses may contain either individual letters or an inclusive range indicated by use of the hyphen (keypunched as minus sign).

In this example, the variables ARROW and TORCH would be recognized as real, DOG and WOLF as integer, and ZEBRA as logical.

Table 23 shows availability of the IMPLICIT statement in various compilers, and also of EQUIVALENCE, discussed in the next section.

The EQUIVALENCE Statement

The specification statement

EQUIVALENCE (ACE,B,CARD)

has the effect of restricting storage reservations to a single location for the variables named. This location will be referenced by *each* of the titles named in the statement. That is, the mention of ACE, B, or CARD would have the same effect at any point in the program, since the location holds only one value. If more than one set of equivalences is to be mentioned, commas are used between separate bracketed sets:

EQUIVALENCE (ACE,B,CARD), (XRAY,ROENT)

The EQUIVALENCE statement is reminiscent of the COMMON statement, which also makes a single storage location accessible by two different titles. Remember, however, that COMMON arranges this location-sharing between variables appearing in different programs or subprograms, while EQUIVALENCE refers to two or more variable titles appearing in the *same* program.

The effect of EQUIVALENCE could be accomplished by actual identical titling of the variables involved, a device that would not have the single-storage effect between main programs and subprograms. EQUIVALENCE is generally used as a convenience in two types of situation. First, it may be used to correct variable title changes that have come about as a result of what the Navy used to call "inadvertence," that is, programmer error. If a variable referred to as WATCH for part of the program has been referred to as CLOCK for other parts, the insertion of

EQUIVALENCE (WATCH,CLOCK)

may be simpler and less error-prone than rewriting and repunching of whole sets of executable statements.

Second, when storage space is tight, further use is made of storage originally reserved for variables needed only in early parts of the execution, by making it available to variables needed only in later portions. For example, suppose that

SUM1, SUM2, SUM3, and SUM4 are needed only until arithmetic means have been computed. The programmer may write

```
----------------
SUM1 = SUM1/150.
SUM2 = SUM2/150.
SUM3 = SUM3/150.
SUM4 = SUM4/150.
------------
```

But then he must remember that from this point in the program "SUM1" is actually an arithmetic mean. The alternative using EQUIVALENCE might read,

```
EQUIVALENCE (SUM1,XM1), (SUM2, XM2), (SUM3,XM3), (SUM4,XM4)
----------------
XM1 = SUM1/150.
XM2 = SUM2/150.
XM3 = SUM3/150.
XM4 = SUM4/150.
```

When *subscripted* variables are to be so treated, the usual rule is that the EQUIVALENCE statement mentions only one numerical subscript, to achieve equivalent storage for the entire array. Thus

```
DIMENSION CAR(50), AUTO(50)
EQUIVALENCE (CAR(1),AUTO(1))
```

arranges for complete identity for all like-subscripted members of the arrays; a total of 50 locations are used.

Order of Specification Statements

For most compilers, all specification statements must precede executable statements of the program. Furthermore, many compilers require a particular order of the specification statements used. The following order is generally acceptable:

Type Statements (REAL, INTEGER, DOUBLE PRECISION,
    COMPLEX, LOGICAL, IMPLICIT)
EXTERNAL
DIMENSION
COMMON
EQUIVALENCE
Statement Function Definitions

Other FORMAT Notations: P, G, and T

The *scale factor* (P) is a method of specifying a shift of the decimal point during input or output of real values (applicable therefore only to F, E, or D specifications). For example, if X is in storage as 1234.5678, the use of the scale factor in *output* causes the following conversions:

Specification	Output
F14.4	1234.5678
0PF14.4	1234.5678
1PF14.4	12345.6780
3PF14.4	1234567.8000
-2PF14.4	12.3456
-4PF14.4	0.1234

Thus "1P" in front of an *output* specification calls for a shift of the decimal point one place to the right; "-1P" shifts the decimal to the left.

Three important points should be noted. First, the appearance of the scale factor in any FORMAT statement is assumed to apply to *all* F, E, and D specifications that follow in the same statement, unless another scale factor cancels the effect. Thus

```
          WRITE (2,10) A, B
   10     FORMAT (2PF14.4,0PF14.4)
```

would result in a shift of the decimal for A and avoid the shift for B.

Second, the application to E notation does not actually change the size of the number, since it changes both position of the decimal *and* the size of the exponent:

```
          C = 1234.5678
          WRITE (2,11) C, C
   11     FORMAT (E16.8/2PE16.8)
```

produces

```
          .12345678E+04
          12.345678E+02
```

both of which have the same value.

Third, the conversion on *input* is in the opposite direction from the output effect. Thus a data item 1234.5678 that the programmer wants to store as 123456.78 would be read according to the instructions,

$$\text{READ (2,12) A}$$
$$\text{12 \quad FORMAT } (-2\text{PF14.4})$$

For both input and output use, therefore, the rule is that

$$\text{external value} = \text{internal value} \times 10^n$$

where nP is used in front of the F specification.

Some compilers provide a *general* specification (symbol G), which may be substituted for F, E, I, D, or L, to describe a data item in terms of (*a*) total width of field "w" and (*b*) total number of digits "d," rather than specifying the precise number of *decimal* locations. The advantages of

$$n\text{Gw.d}$$

are:

1. It will serve for values in any of the five forms for which it substitutes; thus

$$\text{13 \quad FORMAT (G12.5)}$$

might be used in conjunction with

$$\text{WRITE (2,13) A, K, V, BOY}$$

in which A is *real*, K *integer*, V *double precision*, and BOY *logical*. Each variable would occupy 12 total spaces, and up to five characters of each would be produced in output. For example,

$$123.45$$
$$1426$$
$$1.2468$$
$$\text{F}$$

2. The G specification allows the programmer to predetermine the *number of digits* in output of real values, regardless of the predecimal size of the numbers in storage. For instance, if A in the first example had been stored as 1.2345678, the output would still contain five digits:

$$1.2345$$

A "T" specification in FORMAT provides a direct alternative to the "nX" specification. That is, the meaning of

$$\text{T10}$$

is that the *transfer* of data (from input to storage or from storage to output) is
to begin at the *tenth* column. Therefore, the equivalent is

$$9X$$

For example, from this data card:

HARRIS CO. 12500

READ (2,14) PROFIT
14   FORMAT(T11, F6.0)
----

would have the same effect as

READ (2,14) PROFIT
14   FORMAT (10X, F6.0)

However, the "T" notation would also permit READ and WRITE operations
to depart from the usual left-to-right order (which nX cannot accomplish).
This may be illustrated by reading the sample data card in reverse field order:

READ (2,14) PROFIT, FIRM
14   FORMAT (T11, F6.0, T1, A10)

Table 24 shows availability of the P, G, and T FORMAT notations, in
various FORTRAN compilers.

TABLE 24

P, G, and T FORMAT Notations

	P Notation		G Notation		T Notation	
	Yes	No	Yes	No	Yes	No
1[a]		✓		✓		✓
2		✓		✓		✓
3	✓		✓			✓
4	✓			✓		✓
5	✓		✓		✓	
6	✓			✓	✓	
7		✓		✓		✓
8		✓		✓		✓
9	✓			✓		✓

[a] Compiler number.

TABLE 24 (*continued*)

	P Notation		G Notation		T Notation	
	Yes	No	Yes	No	Yes	No
10		✓		✓		✓
11		✓		✓		✓
12		✓		✓		✓
13	✓			✓		✓
14	✓		✓			✓
15	✓		✓		✓	
16	✓			✓		✓
17	✓			✓		✓
18		✓		✓		✓
19		✓		✓		✓
20		✓		✓		✓
21	✓			✓		✓
22	✓		✓		✓	
23	✓		✓			✓
24	✓		✓			✓
25		✓		✓		✓
26	✓		✓			✓
27		✓	✓			✓
28		✓		✓		✓
29	✓		✓		✓	
30	✓			✓		✓
31	✓			✓		✓
32		✓		✓		✓
33	✓		✓			✓
34	✓		✓			✓
35		✓	✓			✓
36	✓		✓			✓
37	✓		✓			✓
38	✓		✓			✓
39	✓			✓		✓
40	✓			✓	✓	
41		✓		✓		✓
42	✓		✓		✓	
43	✓		✓		✓	
44		✓		✓	✓	
45	Output only			✓		✓

TABLE 24 (*continued*)

	P Notation		G Notation		T Notation	
	Yes	No	Yes	No	Yes	No
46	Output only			✓		✓
47	✓			✓		✓
48		✓		✓		✓
49		✓		✓		✓
50	✓			✓		✓
51	✓			✓		✓
52	✓			✓		✓
53	✓			✓		✓
54	✓			✓		✓
55	✓			✓		✓
56	✓		✓			✓
57	✓		✓			✓
58	✓			✓		✓
59	✓			✓		✓
60	✓			✓		✓
61	✓		✓			✓
62		✓		✓		✓
63	✓		✓			✓
64	✓		✓		✓	
65		✓		✓		✓
66	✓		✓			✓
67	✓			✓		✓
68	✓		✓			✓
69	✓		✓		✓	
70	✓		✓		✓	
71	✓		✓			✓
72	✓		✓			✓
73	✓			✓		✓
74	✓		✓			✓
75	✓		✓			✓
76	✓		✓			✓
77	✓		✓		✓	
78	✓			✓		✓
79	✓		✓			✓

FORMAT Specifications Treated as Data

We have suggested several types of generality that may be written into programs intended for use as part of a permanent program library. These include methods of avoiding predefinition of the size of the data set, provision of execution-time options, and designation as function or subroutine subprograms. When programs are to be applied to various data sets, and with varying requirements for precise form of output, the FORMAT statement is a frequent bottleneck, since it commits the user to particular forms of input and output records. Some compilers provide a solution, which appears as follows:

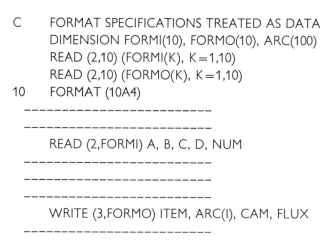

```
C       FORMAT SPECIFICATIONS TREATED AS DATA
        DIMENSION FORMI(10), FORMO(10), ARC(100)
        READ (2,10) (FORMI(K), K=1,10)
        READ (2,10) (FORMO(K), K=1,10)
10      FORMAT (10A4)
        ------------------------
        ------------------------
        READ (2,FORMI) A, B, C, D, NUM
        ------------------------
        ------------------------
        ------------------------
        WRITE (3,FORMO) ITEM, ARC(I), CAM, FLUX
        ------------------------
```

The only FORMAT statement actually written into this source program is one (statement 10) that serves the input statements designed to read FORMAT specifications as *alphameric* data. This statement must specify "A" format. The first arrays (subject to the usual titling conventions) appearing in the DIMENSION statement are designed to store the alphameric characters that make up the *bracketed parts of the missing FORMAT statements* (including left and right parentheses).

The data deck for this example might begin:

(F10.1,E10.0,2F8.4,I10)   (input format for A,B,C,D,NUM)
(1H 4HPAGE,I5,3F12.2)   (output format for ITEM, ARC(I), CAM, FLUX)
   1245.61 1564.E+10. 11.2431 16.4387   (first data)

The first two cards (which must begin with a left parenthesis in column 1) are read in A FORMAT, resulting in storage as follows:

Storage Location	Characters Stored
FORMI(1)	(F10
FORMI(2)	.1,E
FORMI(3)	10.0
FORMI(4)	,2F8
FORMI(5)	.4,I
FORMI(6)	10)
FORMI(7)	
FORMI(8)	
FORMI(9)	
FORMI(10)	
FORMO(1)	(1H
FORMO(2)	4HPA
FORMO(3)	GE,I
FORMO(4)	5,3F
FORMO(5)	12.2
FORMO(6)	)
FORMO(7)	
FORMO(8)	
FORMO(9)	
FORMO(10)	

As you can see, extra space has been provided for larger FORMAT statements. Note that the input and output statements (see the sample program) that use these specifications utilize the subscript-omission method of designating the entire arrays. Also, note that the word "FORMAT" is not read in as data (nor is any statement number for the FORMAT statement).

Table 25 shows availability of this feature, and also of the DATA statement, BLOCK DATA subprogram, and NAMELIST, discussed in succeeding sections.

TABLE 25

FORMAT as Data—Data Initialization—NAMELIST—Holerith Constant

	FORMAT as Data		Data Initialization			NAMELIST		Hollerith Constant	
	Yes	No	DATA	BLOCK DATA	None	Yes	No	Yes	No
1[a]		√			√	√			√
2		√			√	√			√
3	√		√	√		√		√	

[a] Compiler number.

TABLE 25 (*continued*)

	FORMAT as Data		Data Initialization			NAMELIST		Hollerith Constant	
	Yes	No	DATA	BLOCK DATA	None	Yes	No	Yes	No
4		✓	✓	✓			✓	✓	
5	✓		✓	✓		✓		✓	
6	✓		✓				✓		✓
7		✓			✓		✓		✓
8	✓				✓		✓		✓
9	✓		✓b				✓	✓	
10	✓		✓	✓			✓		✓
11	✓		✓b				✓	✓c	
12		✓			✓		✓		✓
13	✓		✓b				✓	✓	
14	✓		✓	✓			✓	✓	
15	✓		✓	✓		✓		✓	
16	✓				✓		✓	✓	
17	✓				✓		✓		✓
18		✓			✓		✓		✓
19		✓			✓		✓		✓
20		✓			✓		✓		✓
21	✓		✓	✓			✓	✓	
22	✓		✓	✓		✓		✓	
23	✓		✓	✓			✓	✓	
24	✓		✓	✓			✓	✓	
25		✓			✓		✓		✓
26		✓			✓		✓		✓
27	✓		✓				✓	✓	
28		✓			✓		✓		✓
29	✓		✓	✓		✓		✓b	
30		✓			✓		✓		✓
31	✓				✓		✓		✓
32		✓			✓		✓		✓
33	✓		✓				✓	✓	

b Data statement uses "=". May be used for labeled common storage.
c Must be declared by "TYPE CHARACTER."

TABLE 25 (*continued*)

	FORMAT as Data		Data Initialization			NAMELIST		Hollerith Constant	
	Yes	No	DATA	BLOCK DATA	None	Yes	No	Yes	No
34	✓		✓	✓		✓		✓	
35		✓			✓		✓		✓
36	✓				✓		✓		✓
37	✓		✓				✓	✓	
38	✓		✓	✓			✓	✓	
39	✓		✓	✓			✓	✓	
40		✓			✓		✓		✓
41		✓			✓		✓		✓
42	✓		✓	✓		✓		✓	
43	✓		✓	✓		✓			✓
44		✓	✓				✓	✓ [d]	
45		✓			✓		✓		✓
46		✓			✓		✓		✓
47	✓		✓				✓	✓	
48		✓			✓		✓		✓
49		✓	✓				✓	✓	
50		✓			✓		✓		✓
51	✓				✓		✓		✓
52	✓		✓	✓			✓	✓	
53		✓			✓		✓	✓	
54		✓			✓		✓		✓
55	✓		✓	✓		✓		✓	
56	✓		✓	✓			✓	✓	
57		✓			✓		✓		✓
58		✓			✓		✓		✓
59		✓			✓		✓		✓
60	✓		✓	✓			✓	✓	
61	✓		✓	✓			✓	✓	
62		✓			✓		✓		✓
63	✓		✓	✓		✓		✓	

[d] Literal only.

TABLE 25 (*continued*)

	FORMAT as Data		Data Initialization			NAMELIST		Hollerith Constant	
	Yes	No	DATA	BLOCK DATA	None	Yes	No	Yes	No
64	√		√	√		√		√	
65		√			√		√		√
66	√		√	√			√	√	
67		√	√				√	√	
68	√		√	√		√		√	
69	√		√	√		√		√ *d*	
70	√		√	√		√		√ *d*	
71	√		√	√			√	√	
72	√		√	√			√	√	
73	√		√	√			√	√	
74	√		√	√			√	√	
75		√	√	√			√	√	
76	√		√	√			√	√	
77	√		√	√		√		√	
78	√		√	√			√	√	
79	√		√	√			√	√	

The DATA Initialization Statement

The following program begins by placing in storage 15 values. (In this instance, the first five are intended as permanent constants, while the next ten are for initialization of sums.)

```
    DIMENSION SUM(10)
    PI = 3.1416
    Z95 = 1.96
    Z99 = 2.58
    ZT95 = 1.64
    AT99 = 2.33
  ┌ DO 1 K = 1,10
1 └ SUM(K) = 0.0
```

The DATA statement offers an alternative method for entering such values into the referenced storage areas.

```
DIMENSION SUM(10)
DATA PI,Z95,Z99,ZT95,ZT99,SUM/3.1416,1.96,2.58,1.64,2.33,10*0.0/
```

This segment replaces all of the previous example. The DATA statement might also have been written

```
DATA PI/3.1416/,Z95,Z99/1.96,2.58/,ZT95,ZT99/1.64,2.33/,SUM/10*0.0/
```

or, if you get the idea, in several other ways as well.

Note that subscripts are omitted in the DATA statement, when full arrays are mentioned. If individual members of arrays are to be treated, the subscript is indicated:

```
DATA SUM(3)/4.6/
```

The indexed-list method is also available within the DATA statement. For example,

```
DATA (NEWS(K),K=1,16)/16*350/
```

The integer constant and asterisk that indicate repetition of a data value may also be used with nonsubscripted variables. Thus

```
DATA F,G,H,I/3*12.0,17/
```

is valid. The statement shown initializes F, G, and H as 12.0, and I as 17.

What is the advantage of entering numerical constants in this manner, rather than by using arithmetic statements that define the values? It is important to observe that the arithmetic-definition method fills locations only during *execution*, while the DATA statement does the job during *compilation*. But it is not execution time that the programmer is trying to save; it is *storage space*. For the statement

$$PI = 3.1416$$

must be translated during compilation to a machine language instruction, which itself takes up core storage space, as part of the object program. This space is in addition to the reserved locations for the variable PI and the constant 3.1416. When the DATA statement is used, the numerical values listed are put directly into appropriately labeled portions of the object program itself (and directly into storage when the object program is loaded), with the result that machine language instruction space is saved.

The initial values thus provided may be changed later in the program (by executable statements); but the DATA statement may not be used to cause reinitialization, since it is not executable. Thus there can be no transfer ("branch") to the DATA statement.

Some compilers (see Table 25) permit initialization of *Hollerith constants* in the DATA statement. This provides a convenient alternative to reading alphameric values as data (using "A" FORMAT). For example, the following program segments accomplish identical storage of the four variables named.

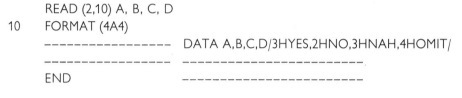

```
        READ (2,10) A, B, C, D
   10   FORMAT (4A4)
        ------------------    DATA A,B,C,D/3HYES,2HNO,3HNAH,4HOMIT/
        ------------------    ------------------------.
        END                   ------------------------
```

(data)   YES NO   NAH OMIT

Some techniques utilizing the DATA statement for Hollerith constants are illustrated in Chapter 13.

The BLOCK DATA Subprogram

Data may *not* be entered into areas of *blank* COMMON by use of the DATA statement. This restriction does not apply to *labeled* COMMON; but the use of the DATA statement to store values in labeled COMMON areas requires a complete subprogram, which may contain *only specification* statements. The subprogram begins with a BLOCK DATA statement:

```
        BLOCK DATA
        DOUBLE PRECISION X(25)
        COMMON /NUM1/K,L,M/NUM2/X
        DATA K,L,M/10,100,1000/,X/25*1.D+12/
        END
```

In this unusual type of subprogram, RETURN is not legal, nor is any other *executable* statement. The subprogram is not *called* by any main program; it is compiled with the main program. We may also observe that this creates one of the rare uses for *labeled* COMMON. Availability of BLOCK DATA is indexed in Table 25.

The NAMELIST Statement

We come finally to a nonexecutable statement that invokes a rather novel method of reading and writing data and is not recommended in ordinary circumstances. The ratio of complex usage rules to actual usefulness is rather high, and omission from most compilers renders programs using NAMELIST nontransferable to many computers.

The statement itself assigns labels to groups of variables, looking very much like the labeled COMMON statement:

NAMELIST /FIRST/A,B,C,D/LAST/E,F,G,H,I,J

The input and output statements that refer to the NAMELIST variables do so by using an equipment unit number in the usual position, and a NAMELIST name in the position usually occupied by a FORMAT statement number. No input or output list is used:

READ (2,FIRST)

WRITE (3,LAST)

The complications arise in preparation of input data.

1. All data cards (or other records) begin in column 2.

2. The ampersand (&) must be used on the first card (record), preceding the NAMELIST name; no data appear on this card.

3. The data set ends with a card (record) containing only the ampersand and the word END.

4. Each data item must be preceded by the appropriate variable title and an equal-sign. An exception permits an array name (written without subscript) to be followed by a series of values separated by commas. If all members of the array are to receive the same value, the n*i form may be used (e.g., M = 10*75, where M is an array dimensioned for ten values).

5. The variables need *not* appear in the same order as they do in the NAMELIST statement. Furthermore, data need not appear for every variable listed in NAMELIST.

6. Each data item must be followed by a comma.

7. Mode conversion takes place as it does in arithmetic statements. Thus A = 12 results in storage of a real value, while I = 6.8 would be stored as 6.

As an example, this program segment

```
DIMENSION PLANT(12), SUM(3), K(5)
NAMELIST /FIRM1/PRICE, QUANT, PLANT, SUM, A, B, C, K
READ (2,FIRM1)
------------
```

might be used in conjunction with this data:

```
&FIRM1
PLANT = 12*1000, PRICE = 6.75, QUANT = 7400,
SUM = 0.0, 4.5, 7.5, K(1) = 20,
A = 10, B = 20,
&END
```

When a NAMELIST name is mentioned in an output statement, output will contain all the significant digits stored for each variable (since no FORMAT statement applies).

Availability of NAMELIST is indexed in Table 25.

For Review	Examples
Specification statement	REAL
	INTEGER
(type specifications)	DOUBLE PRECISION
	COMPLEX
	LOGICAL
	IMPLICIT
	EXTERNAL
	DIMENSION
(storage allocations)	COMMON
	EQUIVALENCE
	DATA
IMPLICIT statement	IMPLICIT INTEGER (A, W−Z)
EQUIVALENCE statement	EQUIVALENCE (WATCH,CLOCK)
G notation	G10.5
P notation (scale factor)	−3PF10.1
T notation	T11
DATA initialization statement	DATA PI/3.1416/,SUM/10*0./,NAME/2HTV/
BLOCK DATA subprogram	
NAMELIST statement	NAMELIST /FIRST/A,B,C,D

	READ (2,FIRST)

EXERCISES

104. Write a program that computes and prints the arithmetic mean of n elements of the X array and then produces a table of X, $(X - \overline{X})$, and $(X - \overline{X})^2$. Read the *input FORMAT* for the X values as data (in A FORMAT). Test the program by first reading the data deck as one item per card and then as five items per card (n = 20 in both instances).

105. Insert a *scale factor* in the first input FORMAT statement of your program for Exercise 104, which will effectively multiply the 20 data items by 100 as they are read. Rerun the program, noting the effects on output.

106. Adjust the program in Exercise 105 by inserting an EQUIVALENCE statement, which specifies equivalence for (a) the sum of the X values and the mean of the X values and (b) the X values and the $(X - \overline{X})^2$ values. Study the changes in output that result.

107. A set of university grade records consists of two cards per student. The first contains the student's name (columns 2–15) and the number of courses attempted (columns 19–20). The second contains letter grades (one for each course attempted), each occupying one column.

Write a program to read these records and compute grade-point averages, calculated for each student as

$$\frac{\sum P}{n}$$

where n is the number of courses attempted and P (points) are awarded as follows:

$$A = 4$$
$$B = 3$$
$$C = 2$$
$$D = 1$$
$$F = 0$$

Use the DATA statement, to

(a) initialize $P_1, P_2, \ldots, P_5$ as 4.0, 3.0, 2.0, 1.0, 0.0,
(b) initialize variables GA, GB, GC, GD, and GF as *Hollerith constants* (which will be compared with the grades read in A FORMAT).

Test your program on the following data:

JONES 10
CBCCABCCCD
SMITH 7
AADCFCC

12 • OPERATING SYSTEMS

General Purpose

In Chapter 2 we indicated that the execution of a program written in FORTRAN language requires performance of several operations before and after entry of the source program. A minimal list would include halting of previous computer operations, resetting of internal and external switches, loading of the FORTRAN compiler program, retrieval and/or loading of the object program, commencement of execution, provision of data if required, and retrieval of output.

In addition to these basic tasks, the programmer may wish to arrange for reproduction (by the computer) of the source program, "tracing" of the program during execution, permanent storage of object program, output, or data, loading of programs or data so stored previously, listing of a "symbol table,"[1] reproduction of parts of on-line or off-line storage, and so on.

An *operating system* (also referred to as a *supervisory* or *monitor* program) is a computer program that remains more or less permanently[2] in on-line storage and has the function of performing most or all of the aforementioned mechanical tasks, and others as well.

Since our viewpoint is that of the FORTRAN language user, rather than the computer center staff, we shall not attempt a complete discussion of the various jobs performed by operating systems. (For example, the supervisory program may perform accounting functions for computer use records, assign or interpret job priorities, allocate time between various remote terminals, and so on.)

Another limitation on our discussion follows from the fact that operating systems differ from computer to computer to a much greater extent than do FORTRAN language compilers. Instead of tabulating control instructions for

---

[1] "Tracing" and "symbol table" will be explained shortly.

[2] In most systems, it may be removed or altered, but not by programmers writing in FORTRAN.

various systems, as we have done for FORTRAN statements, we shall examine one system (IBM 1130) as an example of the requirements and options commonly found in operating systems.

Within this framework, we shall concentrate on those instructions that most frequently precede and follow FORTRAN source programs. Where an operating system is in use, the inclusion of such instructions before and after the source program permits immediate "stacking" of the entire package with a batch of "jobs," which may be run in sequence ("batch-processed") without operator interference.

```
// JOB
// FOR
*IOCS (CARD, 1132 PRINTER, KEYBOARD, TYPEWRITER, DISK)
*NAME MULCO
*EXTENDED PRECISION
**EXERCISE PROBLEM NO. 75 — MULTIPLE CORRELATION
*LIST SOURCE PROGRAM
*LIST SYMBOL TABLE
*LIST SUBPROGRAM NAMES
*ARITHMETIC TRACE
*TRANSFER TRACE
C     (SOURCE PROGRAM BEGINS HERE)
      ------------------
      ------------------
      ------------------
      ------------------
      ------------------
      END
// DUP
*STORE     WS  UA   MULCO
// XEQ MULCO
      -----(Data)--------
      ------------------
      ------------------
      ------------------
      ------------------
```

Essential Control Cards

In this system, only five of these instructions are necessary for *compilation and execution* of the source program:

1. // JOB indicates the beginning of a new job (causing halting of previous operations, resetting of switches, etc.).

2. // FOR causes the FORTRAN compiler program to be transferred into primary storage (from a magnetic disk).

3. *IOCS (abbreviation for Input/Output Control System). The IBM 1130 system requires specification in this form of the input and output equipment that will be used during compilation and execution.

4. *NAME MULCO provides a title by which the program may be referenced, if it is to be permanently stored (as object program).

5. // XEQ causes the object program to be transferred into primary storage and executed. (The invented title "MULCO" need not appear, if // XEQ follows the END statement. In this example, however, the object program has been permanently stored, just prior to execution.)

The control card that specifies EXTENDED PRECISION causes all real variables to be stored in extra-long[3] locations. This substitutes for the DOUBLE PRECISION declaration, which is not available in the 1130 FORTRAN compiler.

Output of Technical Information

The next six instructions call forth extra information as output (beyond the usual error messages and end-of-compilation message).

1. The double-asterisk card provides header information, which will be reprinted at the top of each compilation output page. Since the system is designed for batch processing, such information is convenient for proper separation and allocation of output among the various program authors.

2. The next card calls for reproduction of the source program, as it is read in.

3. The *symbol table* consists of all variable names, statement numbers, statement function names, and constants appearing in the source program, each listed with its address in storage, as assigned during compilation. The table provides a technical aid in debugging and altering programs.

4. The next card calls for a listing of all *subprogram* names mentioned in the source program. This listing serves as a reminder of which subprograms must be in storage when the object program is executed.[4]

---

[3] Three "words" instead of two.

[4] In the 1130 system, source program, symbol table, and subprogram names may all be called for by a single control card, *LIST ALL, which would substitute for the three cards shown.

5. *Arithmetic tracing* is a device used as an aid when "debugging" a program in which errors appear to exist that are difficult to locate by other means. The process consists of printing as output, during execution, the immediate result of *each* arithmetic statement in the source program. That is, each value generated to represent a variable title to the left of an equal-sign will be reproduced as it is transferred to the appropriate storage location.[5]

6. The *transfer trace*, used also for the purpose of debugging, calls for printing of (*a*) each computed value of the expressions within parentheses of IF statements and (*b*) the value of the index variable, for each execution of Computed GO TO statements. (The 1130 system identifies the three trace results as follows:

Arithmetic:	preceded by *
IF:	preceded by **
Computed GO TO:	preceded by ***)

Program Storage

The two control cards following END are designed to effect permanent storage (on magnetic disk) of the *object program* generated by the compilation process:

1. // DUP calls for transfer into storage of a *disk utility program*, which interprets and carries out instructions on "housekeeping" jobs involving transfer of programs and data between disk and input/output media, and between various sections of disk storage. This card is necessary here in order that the next card ("STORE") may be properly interpreted.

2. The "STORE" instruction says, "Transfer the object program from *working storage* to *users' area*[6] (temporary and semipermanent disk storage

---

[5] In the IBM 1130 system, two methods of limiting the trace thus called for are available: (*a*) console entry switch 15 must be ON for trace to be performed, (*b*) tracing may be restricted to parts of the program, by placing the statement CALL TSTOP ahead of segments that are not to be traced and CALL TSTRT ahead of those portions that are to be traced. These options also apply to *transfer trace*.

[6] The "from" initials (WS) appear in columns 13 and 14, the "to" initials (UA) in columns 17 and 18, and the program name in columns 21 to 25. Other abbreviations and meanings in the system include:

PR	PRINCIPAL PRINTING DEVICE
CD	CARD READER
PT	PAPER TAPE
FX	FIXED AREA OF THE DISK

areas); the title MULCO will be used to refer to the program in storage. The purpose is preservation of the object program for future use. For example, the next usage may be accomplished by the following very short set of instructions:

```
//JOB
//XEQ MULCO
------(Data) -----
---------------
---------------
```

If the source program being compiled is actually a *subprogram*, the assigned name must agree with that used in the SUBROUTINE or FUNCTION definition statement and the *NAME control card need not be used. Once stored in this fashion, a subprogram is automatically called by using a proper calling statement in any main program or in any other subprogram.

When main program and subprogram(s) are compiled together, three rules apply:

1. The subprogram must be in storage when the main program is *executed*, but need not be in storage when the main program is being *compiled*.

2. The FORTRAN-compiler control card must appear before each program or subprogram, unless no other activity (e.g., program storage via // DUP) has intervened since the last compilation.

3. IOCS (or comparable instructions in other systems) should not appear in subprogram control cards, since the main program always provides this information.

Our Chapter 8 example, with minimal (IBM 1130 system) control cards, should then be prepared for compilation as follows:

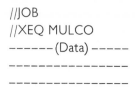

```
// JOB                                          }  control cards
// FOR
        SUBROUTINE PROD
        COMMON F,G,H
        H = F * G                               }  subprogram
        RETURN
        END
// DUP
* STORE    WS  UA  PROD                         }  control cards
// FOR
* IOCS (CARD, 1132 PRINTER, DISK)
```

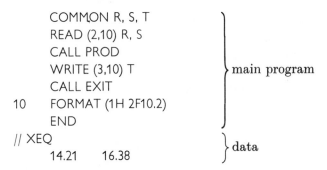

```
        COMMON R, S, T
        READ (2,10) R, S
        CALL PROD
        WRITE (3,10) T          } main program
        CALL EXIT
10      FORMAT (1H 2F10.2)
        END
 // XEQ
        14.21    16.38          } data
```

The *deletion* of the subroutine program from the "user's area" of the disk could be accomplished by the following instruction set:

```
        // JOB
        // DUP
        *DELETE       PROD
```

FORTRAN Statements Related to the Operating System

The presence of an operating system presupposes availability of secondary on-line storage. In FORTRAN compilers written for such systems, the use of this storage by the FORTRAN programmer is facilitated by several specialized statements that may appear within source programs.[7] The five statements described below apply to many IBM systems.

1. When a main program is to use *data* stored magnetically, (e.g., on disk) or is to transfer data or answers *to* such storage, the program must contain a specification[8] statement of the form

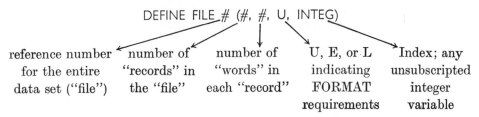

$$\text{DEFINE FILE } \# (\#, \#, U, INTEG)$$

| reference number for the entire data set ("file") | number of "records" in the "file" | number of "words" in each "record" | U, E, or L indicating FORMAT requirements | Index; any unsubscripted integer variable |

---

[7] One statement that we have used earlier, CALL EXIT, is valid only where an operating system is in use. By this time you recognize that it calls a subroutine subprogram stored as part of the operating system. The statement has the effect of returning control to the supervisory program (which then looks for the next // control card).

[8] The statement, when it appears, must precede all statement function definition statements and executable statements.

Since the statement is used only when the program is to read from or write to secondary storage, we defer detailed explanation until these specialized input/ output statements are examined.

2. A statement that transmits a value(s) from primary storage to secondary storage appears in the general form

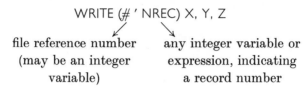

WRITE (# ' NREC) X, Y, Z

file reference number (may be an integer variable) — any integer variable or expression, indicating a record number

Note that the use of the apostrophe in place of the usual comma distinguishes this from an ordinary output statement.

3. The transfer from secondary storage to primary storage is comparable:

READ (# ' NREC) X, Y, Z

The following program segment is designed to read 4000 real data items from cards (they are punched five per card) to secondary storage (via core storage, which could not hold them all at once); and then to bring them back for processing in *reverse* order:

```
10     FORMAT (5F10.4)
       DEFINE FILE 1 (4000,2,U,ITEM)
       ITEM = 1
       DO 11 K = 1,4000,5
       READ (2,10) A1, A2, A3, A4, A5
11     WRITE (1'ITEM) A1, A2, A3, A4, A5
```

```
       DO 21 M = 1,4000
       READ (1'4001 − M) AREA
       VOL = AREA/6. * 3.1416
21
```

The DEFINE FILE statement names the whole data set file number "1," a number that is matched in the READ and WRITE statements referencing this data set. The statement allows for 4000 separate "records," each of which is proper length (two "words," in the IBM 1130 system) for a (single precision) real variable. The "U" signifies "Unformatted," indicating that no FORMAT statements will be used for the transfer of data between primary and secondary storage. Substitution of the letter "E" for "U" would indicate (in some systems) that a FORMAT statement will be required, while the letter "L" leaves the use of FORMAT optional. The FORMAT statement number, when it appears, follows the record-number expression, separated by a comma:

```
        WRITE (1'ITEM,101) A1, A2, A3, A4, A5
101     FORMAT (5F10.4)
```

In the WRITE statement (to the disk, in our example), ITEM is automatically set to the number of the next file record, at the conclusion of each input or output statement using it as an index. This is only true of the index variable mentioned in the original DEFINE FILE statement. Note that initialization is necessary prior to the first usage.

In the READ statement (from the disk; in the second loop) the original index variable is abandoned, since the file is to be read in an order other than record #1 consecutively through record #2000. (Although ITEM is not used by the programmer, it will nevertheless be reset each time the READ statement is executed.)

4.

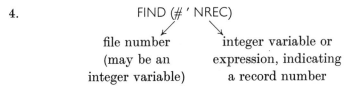

FIND (# ' NREC)

      file number   integer variable or
     (may be an   expression, indicating
  integer variable)   a record number

This statement is inserted to save execution time. It has the effect of moving the necessary physical apparatus ("read-write head") to the secondary storage location specified, in advance of READ or WRITE statements that are going to reference the same area. This movement takes place while other computations are being performed. For example,

```
        _ _ _ _ _ _ _ _ _ _ _ _ _ _ _
        FIND (1'4000)
        _ _ _ _ _ _ _ _ _ _ _ _ _ _ _
        _ _ _ _ _ _ _ _ _ _ _ _ _ _
        _ _ _ _ _ _ _ _ _ _ _ _ _ _
        _ _ _ _ _ _ _ _ _ _ _ _ _ _ _
        DO 21 M = 1,4000
        READ (1'4001 — M) AREA
        _ _ _ _ _ _ _ _ _ _ _ _ _
        _ _ _ _ _ _ _ _ _ _ _ _ _ _
        _ _ _ _ _ _ _ _ _ _ _ _ _
21      _ _ _ _ _ _ _ _ _ _ _ _ _ _
```

5. If two or more main programs are to be used successively for a continuous problem solution, it is convenient to be able to load the second, third, and so on, into core storage without destroying certain values already generated by the earlier programs. If these values are mentioned in COMMON statements within each of the programs, this may be accomplished by

CALL LINK MULCO

⌐ title of the next program,
which is in secondary storage

This appears (it is an executable statement) in the program to be used just prior to MULCO. In many systems, the same effect is achieved by CALL CHAIN.

This feature becomes essential when a program has been written that is too large for the computer system's primary storage. Such a program may be broken into logical "links," each of which fits into primary storage.

For Review	Examples
operating system	
supervisory program	
monitor program	
batch processing	
control cards	// FOR
	*LIST SOURCE PROGRAM
symbol table	
arithmetic trace	
transfer trace	
disk utility program	// DUP
	*STORE WS UA MULCO
working storage	
users' area	
DEFINE FILE statement	DEFINE FILE 1 (4000,2,U,ITEM)
secondary storage WRITE statement	WRITE (1'ITEM) A, B
secondary storage READ statement	READ (1'ITEM) A, B
FIND statement	FIND (1'ITEM)
program links	CALL LINK MULCO

EXERCISES

Note: For each of the programs below, obtain and study available technical output (symbol table, subprogram names). Use arithmetic trace and transfer trace if necessary.

108. When two variables, one of which is categorical and the other quantitative in form, are to be tested for relationship using sample data, the appropriate test is *analysis of variance*. Observations of the quantitative variable fall into as many columns as there are categories of the second variable. These columns will be referred to as a, b, c, etc. The $N_a, N_b, N_c, \ldots$ refer to the numbers of observations in each column. The C will represent the number of columns and N the total number of observations (i.e., $N = N_a + N_b + N_c \cdots$).

Write a program to perform the variance analysis for up to five columns, each with a maximum of 100 observations. The program should read C, N_a, $N_b, N_c, \ldots$ as parameters, compute a sum

$$S = \frac{(\sum X_a)^2}{N_a} + \frac{(\sum X_b)^2}{N_b} + \frac{(\sum X_c)^2}{N_c} + \cdots$$

and then produce as output:

(a) Between-column variance, from

$$BCV = \frac{S - \frac{(\sum X)^2}{N}}{C - 1}$$

(b) Within-column variance, from

$$WCV = \frac{\sum X^2 - S}{N - C}$$

(c) The F ratio, from

$$F = \frac{BCV}{WCV}$$

(d) A statement of the "degrees of freedom," which are

$$(C - 1) \quad \text{and} \quad (N - C)$$

Use your SUMSQ and SQSUM function subprograms (Exercise 98), which should make the variance analysis shorter and easier. Test your program by treating the data deck as a four-column problem, keypunched in column order, $N_a = 20$, $N_b = 25$, $N_c = 30$, $N_d = 25$.

109. Write a program that performs a *frequency count*, producing as output 12 frequencies, representing the classes

$$X < 0$$
$$0 < X < 10$$
$$10 < X < 20$$
$$20 < X < 30$$
$$- - - - - - - - - - -$$
$$90 < X < 100$$
$$X \geq 100$$

Test your program on the entire 100-item data deck.

110. Write a program that will perform *seasonal variation* analysis. The program should read n years of *monthly* data and produce a set of monthly *seasonal indexes*, by the *ratio-to-moving-average* method. The first step is production of a 12-month moving average for the entire series. Since the values of the moving average must be centered, this is followed by a two-period moving average of the first moving average.

   The original monthly values are then expressed as relatives of the moving averages centered opposite them. The seasonal relatives for all Januaries are averaged (arithmetic mean), as are those for all Februaries, Marches, etc.

   Finally, the 12 "seasonal indexes" that result from this process are adjusted so that their sum is equal to 12.00000; the method of adjustment is multiplication of each index by

$$\frac{12.0}{\text{sum of unadjusted indexes}}$$

Test your program by treating the *absolute values* of the first 72 items of the data deck as six years of monthly observations.

13 • SOME PROGRAMMING TECHNIQUES

Having completed your study of FORTRAN language rules, and practiced with each of the permissible statement forms, you should now be adept at translating from problem to computer program. You have seen that there is no single "correct" FORTRAN translation for any real problem; that in fact it is unlikely that any two programmers would ever produce identical programs for the same job. For FORTRAN is truly a language and, like any language, may be used to produce routine prose or ingenious essay. Proust, Camus, and a first-year French student would not produce like responses to the problem of describing their summer vacations, even if their itineraries were identical.

Since there are thus a great variety of "solutions" to each programming problem, we do not propose to end your study with any general presentation of sample programs. However, certain specialized techniques are worthy of note because they are useful in a wide range of problem areas.

Iterative Solutions

The equation

$$X^5 - X^3 = 500$$

may be solved for X, but there is no simple algebraic method for the solution. An *iterative* solution (which might appropriately be defined as "trial-and-error") is begun as follows:

1. Convert to

$$X^5 - X^3 - 500 = 0$$

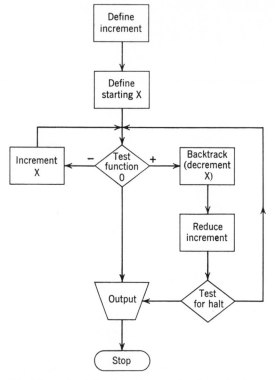

FIG. 15 Flow chart for iterative evaluation of a function.

2. Calculate for various trial values:

Trial Value for X	X^5	X^3	$X^5 - X^3 - 500$
1.0	1.00	1.00	-500.00
2.0	32.00	8.00	-476.00
3.0	243.00	27.00	-284.00
4.0	1024.00	64.00	$+460.00$
3.1	286.29	29.79	-243.50
3.2	335.54	32.77	-197.23
3.3	391.35	35.94	-144.59
3.4	454.35	39.30	-84.95
3.5	525.22	42.88	-17.66
3.6	604.66	46.66	$+58.00$
3.51	532.76	43.24	-10.48
3.52	540.40	43.61	-3.21
3.53	548.12	43.99	$+4.13$
3.521	etc.	etc.	etc.
etc.	etc.	etc.	etc.

All of the work shown produces an answer that is accurate to only one decimal place: 3.5. To fill in three more places (3.5244) the work must be extended proportionally. The process is time-consuming, laborious, and subject to error—a perfect exercise for the computer.

The problem may be verbally summarized thus: start with a trial value of X and evaluate the function $(X^5 - X^3 - 500)$. If the value is *negative*, try a larger X. (A *zero* value would indicate that the trial X is precisely correct; print it.) When this process produces a *positive* value for the function, (*a*) decrease the trial X to its previous (negative-producing) value, (*b*) reduce the increment (to $1/10$ its former size), and (*c*) start the evaluation-increment process again. We should also arrange for a stopping point, when a satisfactory number of decimal places have been computed.

A flow chart diagramming these instructions appears in Fig. 15.

To produce four accurate decimal places, five should be computed. Therefore we shall stop the process when a positive result has been reached with the increment .00001. The program reads:

```
C  ITERATIVE SOLUTION
        REAL INCR
        INCR = 1.0
        X = 1.0
C  EVALUATE FUNCTION
1        IF (X**5 − X**3 − 500.) 2, 5, 3
C  INCREMENT TRIAL VALUE
2        X = X + INCR
        GO TO 1
C  DECREMENT TRIAL VALUE
3        X = X − INCR
C  TEST FOR HALT
        IF (INCR − .00001) 5, 5, 4
C  REDUCE INCREMENT
4        INCR = INCR * .1
        GO TO 2
C  OUTPUT SOLUTION
5        WRITE (3,6) X
6        FORMAT (F15.5)
        CALL EXIT
        END
```

The method has general applicability for iterative problems. For example, if no square root function were supplied by the FORTRAN compiler, we could write one using the same technique:

```
        FUNCTION SKRT(S)
        REAL INCR
        INCR = 1.0
        SKRT = 1.0
        SQ = S
        IF (S) 7,1,1
7       WRITE (3,10)
10      FORMAT (12H SQRT OF NEG)
        SQ = ABS(S)
1       IF (SKRT * SKRT − SQ) 2,5,3
2       SKRT = SKRT + INCR
        GO TO 1
3       SKRT = SKRT − INCR
        IF (INCR − .00000001) 5,5,4
4       INCR = INCR * .1
        GO TO 2
5       RETURN
        END
```

We have included an error message and conversion to absolute value for negative arguments passed to the subprogram.

Sorting Programs

In Chapters 6 and 7 we looked at two slightly different programs for sorting (or "ranking") values. Many ingenious programs have been devised for performing this job. One of the fastest[1] appears below, written as a subprogram:

```
        SUBROUTINE SORT(N)
        COMMON A(500)
        M = N
20      M = M/2
        IF (M) 30,40,30
30      K = N − M
        J = 1
```

---

[1] Published by Marlene Metzner, Pratt & Whitney Aircraft Company. From a method described by D. L. Shell.

```
41      I = J
49      L = I + M
        IF (A(I) − A(L)) 60,60,50
50      B = A(I)
        A(I) = A(L)
        A(L) = B
        I = I − M
        IF (I − 1) 60,49,49
60      J = J + 1
        IF (J − K) 41,41,20
40      RETURN
        END
```

The argument, N, is the number of elements to be sorted. The resulting order is low-to-high; this may be reversed by rewriting the comparison statement,

$$\text{IF } (A(I) − A(L))\ 50,60,60$$

For 100 items, this method begins by comparing X_1 and X_{51}, X_2 and X_{52}, and so on. Though the logic is more difficult to follow than in the basic versions we looked at earlier, this is impressively faster in execution; and the execution time appears to be a nearly linear function of n, whereas most other methods are closer to exponential in this relationship.

Alphameric Sorting

The usefulness of sorting programs is greatly amplified by the fact that *alphabetic* characters may be sorted by the arithmetic sorting routines—for example, alphabetization may be performed by computer.

This is possible because alphameric characters, which have been read in A format or defined by the use of Hollerith constants in the DATA statement, are actually represented in storage by values that have direct numerical (and incidentally alphabetic) interpretations. For example, the statements

```
      -----------------
      READ (2,10) N1, N2, N3, N4
      WRITE (3,11) N1, N2, N3, N4
10    FORMAT (4A1)
11    FORMAT (1H 4I7)
      -----------------
```

in conjunction with a data card containing

ABCZ

would produce, in some IBM systems,

$$-16064 \ -15808 \ -15552 \ -5824$$

Note that the integer values increase through the alphabet.

We may make use of this information to accomplish alphabetization of n names, each containing a maximum of m characters. Since the sorting will have to be performed m separate times (once for each column), we shall use a sorting routine that does not disturb the order of previous results.[2] Our program in Chapter 7 (Ranking Method 2C) meets this requirement. We make four adjustments to the original program:

1. We provide for integer mode, since we are dealing with integer storage.

2. We use double dimension, which will be conceptually helpful for handling n names ("rows"), each of which contains m characters ("columns").

3. We arrange for m executions of the original sorting routine, and for interchange of all m columns, whenever the storage order is switched. (The sorting is done, as it would be by mechanical means, from right to left, to give precedence to leftmost characters.)

4. The alphameric *blank* has a higher value (+16448) than any letter. Since alphabetization convention requires the opposite (e.g., SPA before SPAN), we test for blanks and change their sign to negative (the first set of loops in the program).

```
         SUBROUTINE ALPHA(N,M)
         COMMON LETT(100,10)
        ┌─DO 30 I = 1,N
        │┌─DO 30 J = 1,M
        ││ IF (LETT(I,J) − 16448)30,31,30
   31   │└─LETT(I,J) = (−LETT(I,J))
   30   └─CONTINUE
         LIM = N − 1
```

---

[2] The Metzner routine might be utilized, but since each sort changes the previous sort-result, the program must be arranged so that 26 separate sorting jobs (one for each letter in the (m − 1)th sort) are performed in all columns after the first.

```
       DO 4 NCOL = 1,M
       CALL SLITE(4)
       ICOL = M + 1 − NCOL
       DO 3 L = 1,LIM
       CALL SLITET(4,INTER)
       GO TO (1,4),INTER
   1   MAX = N − L
       DO 3 J = 1, MAX
       IF (LETT(J,ICOL) − LETT(J+1,ICOL))3,3,2
   2   DO 22 K = 1,M
       SAVE = LETT(J,K)
       LETT(J,K) = LETT(J+1,K)
  22   LETT(J+1,K) = SAVE
       CALL SLITE(4)
   3   CONTINUE
   4   CONTINUE
       RETURN
       END
```

A calling program may then alphabetize 50 cards, 8 columns each, as follows:

```
C      CALLING PROGRAM FOR ALPHA
       COMMON K(100,10)
       READ (2,10) ((K(I,J),J=1,8),I=1,50)
       CALL ALPHA(50,8)
       WRITE (2,10) ((K(I,J),J=1,8),I=1,50)
  10   FORMAT (8A1)
       CALL EXIT
       END
```

Bibliographical Manipulation

The alphabetization problem is drawn from a large and growing computer application field, variously referred to as "linguistic," "biliographical," "content analysis," and so on. Since the computer can, as we have seen, store individual alphabetic characters and strings of such characters as *variables*, it is usable for manipulation and analysis of a completely nonnumeric, or literary, nature. This sort of manipulation is useful in a large range of problems: language translation, index and concordance creation, literary style analysis, authorship determination, information retrieval, cryptography, and so on.

The A FORMAT arrangement is the principal FORTRAN tool available for such problems. As an example, let us write a program to read cards on which sentences are punched, and count (a) the number of words and (b) the number of sentences. We shall assume that words are separated by exactly one blank and that the period appears only at the end of a sentence and is followed by one blank before the next sentence begins. The end of the text will be signaled by "/" (separated from the text by a blank column).

```
C       WORD AND SENTENCE COUNT
        DIMENSION LETT(80)
        DATA LPER, LBLANK, LSLASH/1H.,1H ,1H//,NWORD, NSENT/0,0/
1       READ (2,10) LETT
        DO 6 K = 1,80
        IF (LETT(K) − LSLASH)2, 7, 2
2       IF (LETT(K) − LPER) 4, 3, 4
3       NSENT = NSENT + 1
        GO TO 6
4       IF (LETT(K) − LBLANK) 6, 5, 6
5       NWORD = NWORD + 1
6       CONTINUE
        GO TO 1
7       WRITE (3,11) NWORD, NSENT
10      FORMAT (80A1)
11      FORMAT (I6' WORDS'10X,I6' SENTENCES')
        CALL EXIT
        END
```

As an alternative to the DATA statement for initializing Hollerith constants, direct integer assignment could be used (assuming, e.g., the same IBM A1-FORMAT equivalents mentioned earlier):

$$LPER = 19264$$
$$LBLANK = 16448$$
$$LSLASH = 24896$$

Having assigned Hollerith values by either method, the program reads a card, storing each of the 80 characters as a separate array element, and examines them one by one in a loop. The first comparison tests for the "/" and branches to the output statement when it is encountered. The second comparison tests for the period and increases the sentence count when it is found. The third comparison examines for the blank character and upon finding one branches to an increase of the word count. After normal exit from the loop, the unconditional branch leads to input of the next card, which continues the text (which must end in column 80 of each card and begin again in column 1 of the next, even though words are split by the process).

A program using the same general technique performs a word-length analysis, producing as output the number of words found of each length, 1–15:

```
C     WORD LENGTH ANALYSIS
      DIMENSION LETT(80), NUM(15)
      DATA LPER,LBLANK,LSLASH,LCOMMA/1H.,1H ,1H/,1H,/,NUM/15*0/
      KSAVE = 0
I     READ (2,13) LETT
      K = 0
      DO 10 L = 1,80
      IF (LETT(L) − LSLASH) 2, 11, 2
2     IF (LETT(L) − LPER)3, 4, 3
3     IF (LETT(L) − LCOMMA) 5, 4, 5
4     K = K + 1
      KSAVE = KSAVE + 1
      GO TO 10
5     IF (LETT(L) − LBLANK) 10, 6, 10
6     IF (KSAVE − K) 7, 8, 7
7     M = L + 79 − KSAVE
      GO TO 9
8     M = L − K − 1
9     NUM(M) = NUM(M) + 1
      K = L
      KSAVE = K
10    CONTINUE
      GO TO 1
11    DO 12 L = 1,15
12    WRITE (3,14) L, NUM(L)
13    FORMAT (80A1)
14    FORMAT (1H 2I5)
      CALL EXIT
      END
```

In this program, K is used to mark the position of the last blank. When a period or comma (the only clause-ending characters assumed in use) are encountered, K is incremented, to achieve a count adjustment when the following blank is reached. When a blank character is found, the letter count is computed as L-K-1, L being the current blank position and K the prior blank position (or the position to its right, if a punctuation adjustment has been made). An exception is made when the blank is the first one encountered on a continuation card (i.e., when KSAVE ≠ K), to assure counting of the final characters on the preceding card.

Diagram-Producing Programs

For many computer systems, a "plotter" is available—an output device that specializes in graphic representation of functions and/or specific coordinate sets. The FORTRAN programmer can arrange graphic output in the absence of such equipment, by utilizing the FORTRAN language features that we have discussed. The major requirements are "A" format, printer carriage control, and a little ingenuity.

Let us design a subprogram that will plot on a rectangular coordinate grid composed of 72 columns (X axis) and 42 print lines (Y axis). This specifies a square grid of about $7\frac{1}{8}$ inches, on most equipment.

To adjust the Y and X values to this 42 × 72 scale, each value must be divided by a factor computed from

$$\frac{\text{actual range}}{\text{grid range}}$$

Assuming prior storage of the two function subprograms referenced, we may obtain:

$$FY = (BIG(Y,N) - SMALL(Y,N))/42.0$$
$$FX = (BIG(X,N) - SMALL(X,N))/72.0$$

and then reduce (or inflate) the actual values by

```
    ┌ DO 1 K = 1,N
    │ Y(K) = Y(K)/FY
  1 └ X(K) = X(K)/FX
```

To use the *asterisk* as a plotting symbol, if the "Hollerith constant" is available, we initialize

DATA NSPOT/1H∗/

Alternatively, we may specify the integer (A1 format) equivalent:[3]

NSPOT = 23616

By either method, the result of

WRITE (3,10) NSPOT

10   FORMAT (1H A1)

will be the printing of an asterisk.

Vertical distances (computed as differences between Y values) may be translated to carriage control repetition:

⎡DO 7 J = 1,LYDIF

7   ⎣WRITE (3,1000)

1000   FORMAT (1H)

Horizontal distances (computed as differences between X values and the *smallest* X value) may be translated to the printing of *blank* characters, which first must be stored:

INTEGER BLANK(72)

⎡DO 200 K = 1,72

200   ⎣BLANK(K) = 16448

or, if the Hollerith constant is available,

INTEGER BLANK(72)

DATA BLANK/72∗1H /

With either method, we may then accomplish the printing of an asterisk, at the (LXDIF + 1)th column by:

WRITE (3,1001) (BLANK(K),K=1,LXDIF), NSPOT

Since the printer cannot be vertically reversed (i.e., backspaced upward), it is necessary to treat Y values in order from largest to smallest. Therefore the Y–X pairs must be sorted in descending Y order early in the subprogram. A

---

[3] IBM 1130 computer.

subprogram to accomplish this uses the Metzner method discussed earlier in this chapter:

```
        SUBROUTINE YXSORT(Y,X,N)
        DIMENSION Y(1),X(1)
        M = N
        M = M/2
        IF (M) 30,40,30
30      K = N − M
        J = 1
41      I = J
49      L = I + M
        IF (Y(I) − Y(L))50,60,60
50      B = Y(I)
        Y(I) = Y(L)
        Y(L) = B
C   SWITCH X VALUES ALSO
        B = X(I)
        X(I) = X(L)
        X(L) = B
        I = I − M
        IF (I − 1) 60,49,49
60      J = J + 1
        IF (J − K) 41,41,20
40      RETURN
        END
```

This differs from our SORT subprogram only in the direction of ordering (in this instance, from high to low) determined by the central IF statement and in the inclusion of the companion (X) variable in the storage-exchange section.

The two other subprograms called will be:

```
        FUNCTION BIG(A,N)
        DIMENSION A(1)
        BIG = A(1)
      ┌ DO 1 K = 2,N
      │ IF (A(K) − BIG)1,1,2
2     │ BIG = A(K)
1     └ CONTINUE
        RETURN
        END
```

```
                    FUNCTION SMALL(A,N)
                    DIMENSION A(1)
                    SMALL = A(1)
                   ┌DO 1 K = 2,N
                   │IF (A(K) − SMALL)2,1,1
          2        │SMALL = A(K)
          1        └CONTINUE
                    RETURN
                    END
```

A statement function will be employed for rounding differences to the nearest whole scale value. The diagramming subprogram may now be written as follows:

```
                    SUBROUTINE DIAGR(Y,X,N)
                    INTEGER BLANK(73)
                    DIMENSION Y(1), X(1)
                    ROUND(G) = G + .5 * (G/ABS(G))
                   ┌DO 200 K = 1,73
       2000        └BLANK(K) = 16448
                    NSPOT = 23616
                    FY = (BIG(Y,N) − SMALL(Y,N))/42.
                    FX = (BIG(X,N) − SMALL(X,N))/72.
                   ┌DO 1 K = 1,N
                   │Y(K) = Y(K)/FY
       1           └X(K) = X(K)/FX
                    CALL YXSORT(Y,X,N)
                    XSMALL = SMALL(X,N)
                    YLAST = Y(1)
                   ┌DO 2 M = 1,N
                   │LYDIF = ROUND(YLAST − Y(M))
                   │IF (LYDIF)8,8,6
       6           │┌DO 7 J = 1, LYDIF
       7           │└WRITE (3,1000)
       1000        │FORMAT (1H )
       8           │LXDIF = ROUND(X(M) − XSMALL + 1.0)
                   │WRITE (3,1001) (BLANK(K), K = 1,LXDIF), NSPOT
       1001        │FORMAT (1H+74A1)
       2           └YLAST = Y(M)
                    RETURN
                    END
```

A calling program could plot actual X and Y observations (e.g., for the "scatter diagram" used in correlation analysis) as follows:

```
DIMENSION X(20), Y(20)
READ (2,10) (X(K), Y(K), K = 1,20)
CALL DIAGR (Y,X,20)
```

Plotting of a specific function within a specified range could be arranged as follows (Y = sine X, for X from 0 to 4.9 radians, in increments of .1 radians):

```
    DIMENSION X(50), Y(50)
   ┌DO 1 K = 1,50
   │Z = K − 1
   │X(K) = Z/10.
 1 └Y(K) = SIN(X(K))
    CALL DIAGR (Y,X,50)
```

(A disadvantage of the technique, compared to "plotter" equipment performance, may be observed in the flattening out of the top and bottom of the resulting sine curve. Plotters work in scales as small as .01 inches, while the smallest printer movement is about $1/16$ of an inch).

Simultaneous Linear Equations

The solution of sets of simultaneous equations is a part of problems in many fields, which generated laborious computation in precomputer history. A subprogram that will arrive at solutions for any number of equations (up to some dimensioned maximum) is extremely useful and is also an excellent illustration of the handling of a two-dimensional array.

Three general methods for solution are available: determinants, iteration, and elimination. The latter is familiar to most students and is simpler to program as well as more efficient in execution than are the others. An example of the elimination method for three equations follows:

$$3X + 6Y − 6Z = −27$$
$$2X + 8Y + 4Z = − 2$$
$$4X + 12Y + 8Z = 4$$

As a first step, the first equation is divided by 3, to obtain an X-coefficient of 1:

$$X + 2Y - 2Z = -9$$
$$2X + 8Y + 4Z = -2$$
$$4X + 12Y + 8Z = 4$$

The second and third equations are then transformed by subtracting from each an equation consisting of the first multiplied by the later X-coefficients:

second: $2X + 8Y + 4Z = -2$
subtract: $\underline{2X + 4Y - 4Z = -18}$
$4Y + 8Z = 16$

third: $4X + 12Y + 8Z = 4$
subtract: $\underline{4X + 8Y - 8Z = -36}$
$4Y + 16Z = 40$

We have now eliminated all but one X term:

$$X + 2Y - 2\dot{Z} = -9$$
$$4Y + 8Z = 16$$
$$4Y + 16Z = 40$$

The second equation is now divided by 4 (its new Y-coefficient):

$$X + 2Y - 2Z = -9$$
$$Y + 2Z = 4$$
$$4Y + 16Z = 40$$

And the elimination proceeds:

first: $X + 2Y - 2Z = -9$
subtract: $\underline{2Y + 4Z = 8}$
$X - 6Z = -17$

third: $4Y + 16Z = 40$
subtract: $\underline{4Y + 8Z = 16}$
$8Z = 24$

The elimination has now produced:

$$X - 6Z = -17$$
$$Y + 2Z = 4$$
$$8Z = 24$$

The third equation is now divided by 8:

$$X - 6Z = -17$$
$$Y + 2Z = 4$$
$$Z = 3$$

And the final set of subtractions is based on appropriate multiples of this new third equation:

first: $X - 6Z = -17$
subtract: $\underline{- 6Z = -18}$
$X = 1$

second: $Y + 2Z = 4$
subtract: $\underline{2Z = 6}$
$Y = -2$

The remaining equations give the solutions:

$$X \qquad = \quad 1$$
$$Y \qquad = -2$$
$$Z = \quad 3$$

To generalize this solution method, let us list the computations performed on the original coefficient matrix,

$$
\begin{array}{rrrr}
3 & 6 & -6 & -27 \\
2 & 8 & 4 & -2 \\
4 & 12 & 8 & 4
\end{array}
$$

We shall describe the coefficients as a two-dimensional array, with subscripts as suggested in Chapter 6:

$$
\begin{array}{cccc}
1,1 & 1,2 & 1,3 & 1,4 \\
2,1 & 2,2 & 2,3 & 2,4 \\
3,1 & 3,2 & 3,3 & 3,4
\end{array}
$$

In the following list, we omit all computations that are logically designed to produce results of *zero* or *one*, since these values are not used in succeeding computations.

I. Reduction of the first X-coefficient to 1:

$$(1,2) = (1,2)/(1,1)$$
$$(1,3) = (1,3)/(1,1)$$
$$(1,4) = (1,4)/(1,1)$$

A. Transformation of the second equation to eliminate the X term:

$$(2,2) = (2,2) - (2,1)*(1,2)$$
$$(2,3) = (2,3) - (2,1)*(1,3)$$
$$(2,4) = (2,4) - (2,1)*(1,4)$$

B. Transformation of the third equation to eliminate the X term:

$$(3,2) = (3,2) - (3,1)*(1,2)$$
$$(3,3) = (3,3) - (3,1)*(1,3)$$
$$(3,4) = (3,4) - (3,1)*(1,4)$$

II. Reduction of the second Y-coefficient to 1:

$$(2,3) = (2,3)/(2,2)$$
$$(2,4) = (2,4)/(2,2)$$

A. Transformation of the first equation to eliminate Y:

$$(1,3) = (1,3) - (1,2)*(2,3)$$
$$(1,4) = (1,4) - (1,2)*(2,4)$$

B. Transformation of the third equation to eliminate Y:

$$(3,3) = (3,3) - (3,2)*(2,3)$$
$$(3,4) = (3,4) - (3,2)*(2,4)$$

III. Reduction of the third Z-coefficient to 1:

$$(3,4) = (3,4)/(3,3)$$

A. Transformation of the first equation to eliminate Z:

$$(1,4) = (1,4) - (1,3)*(3,4)$$

B. Transformation of the second equation to eliminate Z:

$$(2,4) = (2,4) - (2,3)*(3,4)$$

The programming job appears to require a nest of four loops. Designating the number of rows (equal to the number of equations and/or unknowns) as NR and defining NC = NR + 1, the outer loop must run from 1 to NR (representing I, II, and III in the outline). We begin:

DO 3 I = 1,NR

The reduction work under I, II, and III begins at the (I + 1)th column and proceeds to the last column. Therefore we continue,

M = I + 1
⌈DO 1 J = M,NC
1 ⌊C(I,J) = C(I,J)/C(I,I)

The work necessary under A and B in the outline suggests a double loop. Since all but the Ith row must be transformed, the outer loop begins

DO 3 J = 1,NR

but is immediately qualified,

IF (J − I) 22,2,22

The transformation work begins at the (I + 1)th column and proceeds to the last column:

22 ⌈DO 2 K = M,NC
2 ⌊C(J,K) = C(J,K) − C(J,I)*C(I,K)

Written as a subroutine subprogram, for a maximum of twenty equations:

```
            SUBROUTINE SOLVE(C,NR)
            DIMENSION C(20,21)
            NC = NR + 1
          ┌─DO 3 I = 1,NR
          │ M = I + 1
          │ ┌─DO 1 J = M,NC
      1   │ └─C(I,J) = C(I,J)/C(I,I)
          │ ┌─DO 3 J = 1,NR
          │ │ IF (J − I)22,2,22
     22   │ │ ┌─DO 2 K = M,NC
      2   │ │ └─C(J,K) = C(J,K) − C(J,I)*C(I,K)
      3   └─└──CONTINUE
            RETURN
            END
```

A calling program might then read,

```
            DIMENSION X(20,21)
            READ (2,11) ((X(I,J), J=1,4),I=1,3)
            CALL SOLVE (X,3)
            WRITE (3,12) (X(I,4),I=1,3)
     11     FORMAT (12F5.2)
     12     FORMAT (1H03F10.2)
            CALL EXIT
            END
```

Note that the solutions are returned to the calling program as $X(I,NC)$; that is, the right-hand column of the transformed matrix contains the required answers.

There is a flaw in the subprogram as written, however. It is possible that during the elimination process one or more of the diagonal elements may become zero. For example, if the second equation of our example were altered,

$$3X + 6Y - 6Z = -27$$
$$2X + 4Y + 4Z = 6$$
$$4X + 12Y + 8Z = 4$$

The first set of subtractions would become

second:	$2X$	$+4Y$	$+4Z$	$=$	6	third:	$4X$	$+12Y$	$+8Z$	$=$	4
subtract:	$2X$	$+4Y$	$-4Z$	$=$	-18	subtract:	$4X$	$+8Y$	$-8Z$	$=$	-36

second: $\quad 0 \quad +8Z = 24$

third: $\quad 4Y +16Z = 40$

leaving the three equations in this form:

$$X + 2Y - 2Z = -9$$
$$8Z = 24$$
$$4Y + 16Z = 40$$

The attempt to reduce the second equation would now result in division by zero.

This problem may be solved by reversing the second and third equations before proceeding:

$$X + 2Y - 2Z = -9$$
$$4Y + 16Z = 40$$
$$8Z = 24$$

Then the reduction of the second equation presents no problem:

$$X + 2Y - 2Z = -9$$
$$Y + 4Z = 10$$
$$8Z = 24$$

And the transformations are

first: $X + 2Y - 2Z = -9$ third: $8Z = 24$

subtract: $ 2Y + 8Z = 20$ subtract: $0 = 0$

$\overline{X - 10Z = -29}$ $\overline{8Z = 24}$

producing:

$$X - 10Z = -29$$
$$Y + 4Z = 10$$
$$8Z = 24$$

Reduction of the third equation leaves:

$$X - 10Z = -29$$
$$Y + 4Z = 10$$
$$Z = 3$$

and the final transformations produce the correct solutions:

first: $X - 10Z = -29$ second: $Y + 4Z = 10$

subtract: $ - 10Z = -30$ subtract: $ 4Z = 12$

$\overline{X = 1}$ $\overline{Y = -2}$

$$X = 1$$
$$Y = -2$$
$$Z = 3$$

Note that the order of results is not changed by the switch of equation positions.

The adjustment of the subprogram to incorporate the procedure produces this version:

```
        SUBROUTINE SOLVE(C,NR)
        DIMENSION C(20,21)
        NC = NR + 1
       ┌─DO 3 I = 1,NR
       │  KEXCH = 1
       │  M = I + 1
   C   │  TEST OF DIAGONAL ELEMENT
   6   │     IF (ABS(C(I,I))−1.E−05)8,8,7
   C   │  REDUCTION OF I-TH EQUATION
   7   │  ┌─DO 1 J=M,NC
   1   │  └─D(I,J) = C(I,J)/C(I,I)
   C   │  ELIMINATION IN OTHER EQUATIONS
       │  ┌─DO 3 J = 1,NR
       │  │  IF (J − I)22,3,22
  22   │  │┌─DO 2 K = M,NC
   2   │  │└─C(J,K) = C(J,K) − C(J,I)*C(I,K)
   3   └──┴─CONTINUE
        RETURN
   C   INTERCHANGE OF EQUATIONS
   8      L = I + KEXCH
   C   TEST FOR EXISTENCE OF L-TH EQUATION
          IF (L − NR)9,9,30
   9      ┌─DO 111 N = I,NC
          │  SAVE = C(I,N)
          │  C(I,N) = C(L,N)
 111      └─C(L,N) = SAVE
          KEXCH = KEXCH + 1
          GO TO 6
   C   FAILURE MESSAGE
  30      WRITE (3,31)
  31      FORMAT (' EQUATIONS CANNOT BE SOLVED BY PROGRAMMED
                                                    METHOD')
        RETURN
        END
```

Exchanges of coefficients begin at the Ith column, since columns to the left have already been reduced to zero. The KEXCH variable is used to provide successive exchanges of Ith and $(I + 1)$th, $(I + 2)$th, and so on, equations, if successive equations with the same zero term are encountered. If an unreduced equation with the required nonzero coefficient cannot be found, the error message results.

In statement 6, why did we not simply say

$$6 \quad \text{IF } (C(I,I))8,8,7?$$

We have observed that binary computers produce rounding error. Therefore the storage location that should logically hold a zero (as the result of computation) may hold some nonzero digits. For example, in an actual computation

$$(-4.) - 3.*(-4./3.)$$

one binary computer produces

$$0.3725290301E-08$$

Though ten-digit precision is presumed for this system, the number

$$.0000000037$$

would be regarded as nonzero if tested directly in an IF statement. Therefore, the equation reversal is conditioned (statement 6) on the presence of any fairly small number, in the diagonal element. (Small elements are undesirable as reduction pivots in any case, and no damage is done by "unnecessary" reversal of equation positions.)

Simulation Problems

The computer is admirably suited to the exploratory problem-solving techniques grouped under the term "simulation" or the subgroup "Monte Carlo methods." Millions of trials (e.g., simulated time periods, events) may be generated with reasonable speed, and the computer may be used to classify and count results as it generates them.

A specialized compiler language (SIMSCRIPT) has been developed for such problems. However, FORTRAN is certainly usable, if the programmer exercises some ingenuity.

An important element in many simulation problems is the generation of "random" numbers. We shall not discuss alternative computer methods for doing this, beyond noting that they all have in common the generation of repeatable *sequences* of digits, which are therefore more properly called "pseudo-random" numbers. That is, the digit strings that are produced are not truly random, since (a) the same strings are reproducible each time the generation routine is used and (b) the string is of finite length and will begin to repeat when this length has been reached.

These drawbacks are also present, however, in random number *tables*, which historically have been the most common random-digit selection method. When such a table is used, these two faults are usually overcome as follows:

1. By selecting a random starting point for each use of the table.

2. By using a table long enough so that specific strings need not be repeated.

Effective random-number function subprograms contain the same provisions. The following example, adapted for the IBM 1130 computer, uses an external switch to select the starting point and produces 8192 numbers (i.e., may be used sequentially 8192 times) before repeating sequences.[4]

```
        FUNCTION RNS(YFL)
        IF (IXX − 3333) 2,1,2
2       IX = 3333
1       IY = IX * 899
        IF (IY) 5,6,6
5       IY = IY + 32767 + 1
6       RAND = IY
        RAND = DRH(RAND/32767. * (YFL + 1.))
        IX = IY
        IF (RAND − YFL) 7,7,1
7       CALL DATSW (3,L)
        GO TO (1,8),L
8       RNS = RAND
        IXX = 3333
        RETURN
        END
```

(The DRH function is the equivalent of AINT).

If data switch 3 is on, numbers generated are not returned to the calling program. Thus the random starting point is selected by commencing execution with this switch on and by turning it off (at a "random" time) a few seconds after main program execution has begun. This subprogram returns a real value

---

[4] This is not long enough for many problems. The same sort of subprogram is frequently available with nonrepeating length of very much greater duration, for example, 10^{38} returned values before repeating sequences.

(truncated; i.e., with zero decimal constant) which lies between zero and the calling statement argument (which must be real and positive).

Some specific useful applications for simulation problems include:

1. Selection of a random point from a space of given size. For example, from a 200 × 300 grid:

```
Y = RNS(20000.)/100.
X = RNS(30000.)/100.
```

These calling statements arrange for two decimal places in each coordinate, with minimum (0.00, 0.00) and maximum (300.00, 200.00).

2. Simulation of random sampling, from a stored population of given size. For example, from a population of 1000 array elements, a sample of 30 may be generated:

```
    DO 1 M = 1,30
    K = RNS(999.) + 1.
1   SUM = SUM + X(K)
```

This permits subscript generation between 1 and 1000 (inclusive). (Zero is a possible returned result from the function subprogram.)

3. Determination of whether an event occurs, given the overall probability of occurrence. For example, for an event with $1/20$ probability of occurrence:

```
P = RNS(19.)
IF (P) 11,6,11
```

Since the subprogram may return values from 0. to 19. inclusive, the probability of 0. is $1/20$. The program branches to statement 6 if the event occurs.

As an example of "Monte Carlo" methods, consider the following problem, which is also capable of direct mathematical solution. What is the average (arithmetic mean) distance from the center, for all points in a rectangle of given size? Let the rectangle be represented as a 100 × 200 grid:

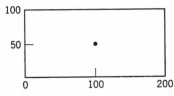

Then the center is at (100, 50).

The following program selects 5000 points at random from within the grid, measures each distance from the center, and computes and prints the mean distance:

```
C       RECTANGLE – DISTANCE SIMULATION
        SUM = 0.
       ┌DO 1 M = 1,5000
       │X = RNS(20000.)/100.
       │Y = RNS(10000.)/100.
    1  └SUM = SUM + SQRT((X−100.)**2 + (Y−50.)**2)
        DMEAN = SUM/5000.
        WRITE (3,10) DMEAN
    10  FORMAT (1H1F10.4)
        CALL EXIT
        END
```

The distance measurement is based on the Pythagorean theorem:

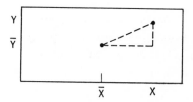

That is, the distance in each case is the hypotenuse of the triangle formed by $(\overline{X}, \overline{Y})$, (X, Y), and $(X, \overline{Y})$ or $(\overline{X}, Y)$.

This example may be extended to solve a problem described as follows: A towing service facility is to be established in a 100 × 200 block area. Frequency of service calls differs in two halves of the area:

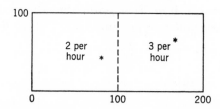

Two locations, (90, 45) and (175, 85), are being considered for the facility. What would be the average distance to accident sites at each location?

The following program simulates 5000 calls to estimate the required averages:

```
C      TOWING SERVICE LOCATIONS
       DIST(A,B) = SQRT((X−A)**2 + (Y−B)**2)
       TOTAL1 = 0.
       TOTAL2 = 0.
       DO 1 M = 1,5000
C   SELECT COORDINATES FOR 100 X 100 HALF-GRID
       Y = RNS(10000.)/100.
       X = RNS(10000.)/100.
C   DETERMINE GRID HALF, USING 2–3 PROBABILITY RATIO
       LOC = RNS (4.) + 1.
       GO TO (2,2,3,3,3),LOC
3      X = X + 100.
2      TOTAL1 = TOTAL1 + DIST(90.,45.)
1      TOTAL2 = TOTAL2 + DIST(175.,85.)
       AVG1 = TOTAL1/5000.
       AVG2 = TOTAL2/5000.
       WRITE (3,10) AVG1, AVG2
10     FORMAT (' LEFT LOCATION'F10.4'RIGHT LOCATION'F10.4)
       CALL EXIT
       END
```

An interesting usage of Monte Carlo methods in mathematics is the estimation of area under a curve, without integration. For example, for the function

$$Y = X^2 - 9$$

what is the area bounded by the curve and the x-axis?

On a graph of the function

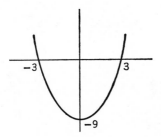

we may superimpose a 9 × 6 rectangle, with total area 54, and write a program

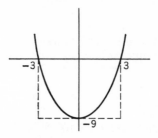

that computes the proportion of (randomly selected) points in the rectangle that fall between the curve and the x-axis, and estimates the required area accordingly.

```
C       AREA BETWEEN Y = X**2 − 9   AND X-AXIS
        UNDER = 0.
        DO 1 M = 1,000
       ┌X = RNS(600.)/100. − 3.
       │Y = RNS (900.)/100. − 9.
       │IF (Y .GT. X**2−9.)   UNDER = UNDER + 1.
1      └CONTINUE
        AREA = UNDER/1000. * 54.
        WRITE (3,10) AREA
10      FORMAT (1H F10.4)
        CALL EXIT
        END
```

The precise answer arrived at by integration is 36.0. The program above, in five separate executions, produced the following results:

1.	34.9380
2.	35.3160
3.	36.1800
4.	37.4760
5.	36.0720
Average	35.9964

For Review

iterative solution
alphameric sorting
A FORMAT integer equivalent

EXERCISES

For Review

elimination method (simultaneous equations)
simulation
Monte Carlo methods
pseudorandom number

EXERCISES

111. *Newton's method* provides a way of finding a root or roots of an equation
$f(x) = 0$. For if x is a root and x_n a nearby value, *Taylor's theorem* provides us
with the approximation

$$f(x) \simeq f(x_n) + (x - x_n)f'(x_n)$$

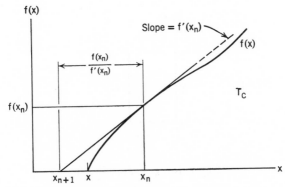

where $f'(x_n)$ is the derivative df/dx evaluated at the point x_n. Since $f(x) = 0$,
if x is a root, we have approximately

$$x \simeq x_n - \frac{f(x_n)}{f'(x_n)}$$

provided that $f'(x_n)$ is not zero. Since the equation is only an approximation,
however, x will not equal the root exactly, but will be a better approximation
than x_n. The process can be repeated, using the calculated value of x as a new
x_n and repeating the calculation. This can be summarized by the iteration
formula

$$x_{n+1} = x_n - \frac{f(x_n)}{f'(x_n)}$$

where the subscript n counts the number of times the iteration has been
repeated. The process is stopped when further repetitions cause the value to
change only insignificantly.

Employ the method to write a function subprogram to find the square root of a number b: $x^2 = b$ or $f(x) = x^2 - b = 0$. Since $f'(x) = 2x$, the iteration formula is

$$x_{n+1} = x_n - (x_n{}^2 - b)/2x_n = (2x_n{}^2 - x_n{}^2 + b)/2x_n = (x_n{}^2 + b)/2x_n$$

Use as an initial guess $x_0 = 1$ and terminate the calculation when successive iterations change the root by less than $b \times 10^{-10}$. Note: are there any values of b that require exceptional treatment?

Test your subprogram by calling it with a program that also uses the SQRT function (Fortran-supplied) and outputs both answers for the argument value.

112. An important problem in quantum mechanics is that of a particle of mass m in a square potential well of depth $-V_0$, width a. The problem is to find the *energy eigenvalues* E of the particle. One finds the latter by solving for the real roots ξ of the transcendental equation

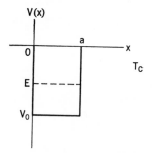

$$f(\xi) = \tan \xi + \xi(b^2 - \xi^2)^{-\frac{1}{2}} = 0$$

where $\xi^2 = -2mEa^2/\hbar^2$, $b^2 = -2mV_0a^2/\hbar^2$ ($2\pi\hbar$ is Planck's constant). Since the equation is an odd function of ξ, we need look only for positive roots. The second term must be real and nonnegative, hence the roots ξ must fulfill the relations (i) $(2m - 1)\pi/2 \le \xi \le m\pi$, where $m = 1, 2, 3, \ldots$; (ii) $\xi \le b$. Condition (ii) means that m cannot exceed $(b/\pi) + \frac{1}{2}$.

Use the *Newton algorithm* discussed in Exercise 111 for improving the approximation to a root:

$$\xi_{n+1} = \xi_n - g(\xi_n) \quad \text{where} \quad g(\xi) = \frac{f(\xi)}{f'(\xi)}$$

For the problem at hand,

$$g(\xi) = \frac{[\xi + (b^2 - \xi^2)^{\frac{1}{2}} \tan \xi](b^2 - \xi^2) \cos^2 \xi}{(b^2 - \xi^2)^{\frac{3}{2}} + b^2 \cos^2 \xi}$$

Note that when an equation has more than one root (as is the case here) the selection of a starting approximation ξ_0 is most critical. From the form of the equation we see that the lowest root lies between $\pi/2$ and the smaller of π and b, the second root between $3\pi/2$ and the smaller of 2π and b, and so forth. So use as a starting value for the mth root

$$\xi_0^{(m)} = \frac{\dfrac{2m-1}{2}\pi + \min(m\pi, b)}{2}$$

Determine all the roots $\xi^{(m)}$ for each of the ten well sizes b $= 1, 2, 3, \ldots, 10$, to an accuracy of 0.01 per cent. For each b, first determine the number of roots, m_{max}. Then calculate the roots $\xi^{(1)}, \xi^{(2)}, \ldots, \xi^{(m_{max})}$.

113. Write a program that will compute and print the *median* of any set of up to 200 values of X, entered in random order; call a *sorting subprogram* to do the ordering. (The median is defined as the $(n+1)/2$th item of an *ordered* array; for even numbers of elements, the median is approximated as the arithmetic mean of the two "middle" elements.) The program should read "n" as a parameter preceding the data. Test your program first on the first 20 data items and then on the first 25 data items.

114. Write a program that will determine the frequency of occurrence of the word "THE" in a group of sentences keypunched on cards. To test your program, keypunch the sentence:

THE USE OF ETHER AS AN ANESTHETIC
MARKED THE BEGINNINGS OF THE
MODERN ERA OF SURGICAL TECHNIQUE.

115. Write a program that will examine a given deck of sentences, to find and reprint all the words that contain three or more vowels. Test your program on the Exercise 114 sentence.

116. To fit a *quadratic curve* ($Y_c = a + bX + cX^2$) by least-squares methods, the following normal equations may be solved for a, b, and c:

$$\sum Y = na + b \sum X + c \sum X^2$$
$$\sum XY = a \sum X + b \sum X^2 + c \sum X^3$$
$$\sum X^2Y = a \sum X^2 + b \sum X^3 + c \sum X^4$$

Write a program that reads n values of X and Y and calls the SOLVE subroutine subprogram (or other subprogram available for simultaneous linear equations), to produce the values of a, b, and c. Test your program on the first 40 data items, treating the first 20 as X values and the next 20 as Y values.

117. The Monte Carlo method of integration becomes really useful when the boundaries are complicated or when the integral has several dimensions. Evaluate the shaded area in the figure below—the area inside a circle of radius

4, but outside an ellipse of semiaxes 3 and 6 and concentric with the circle. The circle's boundary is given by

$$X^2 + Y^2 = 16$$

and that of the ellipse is given by

$$(X/6)^2 + (Y/3)^2 = 1$$

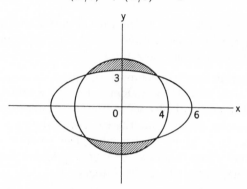

118. Assume a function subprogram in storage, called KRAND, which returns a random *integer* between 1 and K, where K is the integer argument. Write a main program that reads 100 *real* values and then uses the subprogram to select a random sample of 12 of these data items. Output should include all the real values selected for the sample, their array positions, and the sample arithmetic mean.

119. Since the Central limit theorem states that the means of simple random samples are *normally* distributed (around the population mean), a subprogram that returns the *mean* of 30 random numbers would actually be producing "random normal numbers." Write a function subprogram that does so; let it call any simple random number generator available with your system.

120. Write a calling program that selects 500 random normal numbers by utilizing the subprogram in Exercise 119. The calling program should then make a frequency count, using 15 classes with class interval computed as

$$\frac{\text{range of returned values}}{15}$$

Insert an arrangement that calls a diagram-producing subprogram, to "draw" the (normal?) distribution. Use frequencies as Y and class midpoints as X.

appendix A
TEST OUTPUT FOR
EXERCISE PROGRAMS

Use of This Appendix

The output values provided below should be referred to when testing each exercise program. Check carefully, since the absence of compilation error messages signifies correct FORTRAN language, but does not guarantee program logic. You may also find the sample output helpful in clarifying the intent of any program (prior to writing it) for which the problem statement may appear unclear.

There is no single "solution" for any of the exercises; in general, any program that produces the desired output is "correct." However, alternative approaches to a problem may be differentiated on the basis of program length or execution time. Usually, you should aim for the shortest program that will do the job, taking full advantage of each FORTRAN "shortcut" as it is introduced in the text.

Test Data

For exercises requiring data, the sample output results from testing on a standard data set, which should be used for each such problem, unless special data are mentioned in the exercise. The set consists of 20 punched cards (or equivalent records on other input media), coding for which appears in Fig. 16.

Precision of Answers

Since your programs for the first 49 exercises utilize the standard FORMAT statement described in Chapter 2, five decimal places will appear in each output value. Note, however, that differing *precision* limits for real values (indexed in

FORTRAN CODE

alpha 0	= Ø
zero	= O
alpha i	= I
one	= 1
z	= ƶ

FORTRAN CODING FORM

HOFSTRA UNIVERSITY COMPUTER CENTER

PROGRAMMER
PROJECT NUMBER
DATE
Page _____ of _____

FORTRAN STATEMENT — IDENTIFICATION SEQUENCE

19.00	0.04	3.00	5.21	6.00	ALA.
0.04	28.30	19.60	15.00	17.20	ARIZ.
3.00	42.30	0.00	17.00	64.20	ARK.
5.21	47.30	0.00	48.30	20.60	CAL.
6.00	-3.20	-4.21	28.60	27.60	CØL.
0.04	2.45	9.38	9.21	-40.60	CØNN.
28.30	-30.00	7.20	21.20	-20.30	DEL.
19.60	14.60	6.00	28.70	-4.30	D.C.
15.00	93.20	5.70	30.90	9.60	FLA.
17.20	15.80	-4.20	8.70	0.00	GA.
3.00	74.30	-3.80	9.21	28.73	IDAHØ
42.30	61.20	20.60	24.70	-4.30	ILL.
0.00	-28.60	30.00	6.38	9.21	IND.
17.20	12.21	0.00	9.20	8.76	IØWA
64.20	78.40	19.30	-4.20	8.60	KAN.
5.21	-10.12	9.25	6.40	9.75	KY.
47.30	-190.20	-4.30	24.60	0.21	LA.
0.00	1.10.60	8.21	29.90	7.65	MAINE
48.20	74.10	17.20	0.00	8.71	MD.
20.60	60.20	-8.75	6.30	47.20	MASS.

FIG. 16 Standard data set for testing exercise programs.

Table 6) may produce differences in digits at the right of the answer. Answers that agree in the first five or six digits counting from the *left* may be regarded as matching. You should also be aware that the computer may produce "3.99999" when you are expecting the answer "4.00000," as the result of truncation of succeeding digits without rounding. Do not consider discrepancies of such magnitude as evidence of error.

In the first 49 exercises, the fifth decimal digit of the sample output is unrounded, as it would be produced by most FORTRAN compilers. From Exercise 50 forward, answers have been rounded.

1.	1.00000	13.00000
	2.00000	26.00000
	3.00000	39.00000
	4.00000	52.00000
	etc.	

2.	100.00000	161.30000
	110.00000	169.60000
	120.00000	177.90000
	130.00000	186.20000
	etc.	

3.	1.00000	16.08000
	3.00000	144.72000
	5.00000	402.00000
	7.00000	787.92000
	etc.	

4.	10.00000	1707.00000
	20.00000	853.50000
	30.00000	426.75000
	40.00000	213.37500
	etc.	

5.	0.00000	25000.00000	0.00000
	5.00000	20000.00000	112500.00000
	10.00000	15000.00000	200000.00000
	15.00000	10000.00000	262500.00000
		etc.	

6.   4.00000
          2.66666
          3.46666
          2.89523
            etc.

7.   −1.00000   0.76470
         −2.00000   1.52941
         −3.00000   2.29411
         −4.00000   3.05882
                        etc.

8.   12.00000   77.88000   95.76000
         24.00000   155.76000   191.52000
         36.00000   233.64000   287.28000
         48.00000   311.52000   383.04000
                        etc.

9.   5.00000   25.62083
         10.00000   51.24166
         15.00000   76.86250
         20.00000   102.48333
                        etc.

10.   1.00000   1.26582
          2.00000   2.53164
          3.00000   3.79746
          4.00000   5.06329
                        etc.

11.   1.00000   1.00000
          2.00000   2.00000
          3.00000   6.00000
          4.00000   24.00000
          5.00000   120.00000
                        etc.

12.   2.00000   70710.67767
          3.00000   1709.97594
          4.00000   265.91479
          5.00000   87.05505
                        etc.

13.
5.00000	1210.81484
10.00000	1466.07259
15.00000	1775.14246
20.00000	2149.36885

etc.

14.
0.41759
0.35020
0.42057
0.41752
0.41759

etc.

15.
100.00000	2.49377
200.00000	3.52672
300.00000	4.31934
400.00000	4.98754

etc.

16.
0.00500	1.86855	0.03237	1.83618	5.41812
0.01000	1.89690	0.02793	1.86896	5.31197
0.01500	1.92525	0.02350	1.90175	5.20583
0.02000	1.95360	0.01907	1.93453	5.09969

etc.

17.
1.00200
1.00400
1.00802
1.01612

etc.

18.
10.00000	385.00000
20.00000	2870.00000
30.00000	9455.00000
40.00000	22140.00000

etc.

19.
1.39000	4.54802
1.41000	4.59972
1.43000	4.65102
1.45000	4.70190

etc.

20.   10.00000   0.85866
       20.00000   0.59097
       30.00000   0.47835
       40.00000   0.41249
                    etc.

21.   1.00000   135.00000
        2.00000   95.47858
        3.00000   148.35393
        4.00000   288.22018
                    etc.

22.   1.00000   0.00000
        2.00000   0.30103
        3.00000   0.77815
        4.00000   1.38021
                    etc.

23. 1000.00000   0.05000   0.25231
     2000.00000   0.10000   0.35682
     3000.00000   0.15000   0.43701
     4000.00000   0.20000   0.50462

    30000.00000   1.50000   1.38197

24. 0.11258E+16   0.11258E+16

25.   1.64493
        1.64293

26.   2.34738   9.30747

27.   2.34738   9.30747
        5.64344   18.47101
        0.00000   35.23898
        0.00000   31.66080

       20.03322   35.75609

28.   9.00000   15.00000   93.20000
       12.00000   42.30000   61.20000
       15.00000   64.20000   78.40000

29.   19.00000
        19.60000
        15.00000
        17.20000
        42.30000
        17.00000
        64.20000

30.   18.06000   18.48882

31.   5.00000   23.11640
        10.00000   28.12464
        15.00000   34.21792
        20.00000   41.63133
                               etc.

                                         or, in microamperes:

32. 0.00000E 00   0.33344E−08   0.00000   0.00333
    0.10000E+01   0.96133E−06   1.00000   0.96133
    0.20000E+01   0.19336E−05   2.00000   1.93368
    0.30000E+01   0.29196E−05   3.00000   2.91969
    ────────────────────────────   ──────────────────────
    0.50000E+02   0.50012E−04   50.00000   50.01244

33.   7.34666
         2.75000
         4.73666
         3.75000
         ───────
        22.933333

34.   0.00000   0.75493   0.00000
         0.15000   −0.00506   0.01444
         0.30000   −0.00506   0.01368
         0.45000   −0.00506   0.01292
         ───
         3.00000   −0.00506   0.00000

35.   0.10000   0.11088
         0.20000   0.11022
         0.30000   0.10912
         0.40000   0.10760

         2.00000   0.04739

36.   0.00210
       707.50000
        14.10000
         9.07869

        45.94342   1.53122

37.   0.04000   19.00000
         0.04000   28.30000
         3.00000   43.30000
         5.21000   47.30000

        20.60000   60.20000

38. 10017.56779   18.06000   18.48882

39.   1.00000   0.00000   0.84147
         1.10000   0.09531   0.89120
         1.20000   0.18232   0.93203
         1.30000   0.26236   0.96355

         2.00000   0.69314   0.90929

40.   0.69264   0.69314

41.   1000.00000   21882.24993
      2000.00000   25018.01588

     10000.00000   0.00000
     20000.00000   − 59281.58750

    100000.00000   − 691977.50268

    900000.00000   − 8147932.50585

42.   18.06000   18.11233

43.   2.71828   2.71828

44.   39.33988
       0.00000
       1.79175
       4.78749

       42.33561

45. As pictured in exercise.

46.   19.00000
       3.00000
       15.00000
       3.00000
       17.00000

47.   50.00000   3.68403
       55.00000   3.80295
       60.00000   3.91486
       65.00000   4.02072

       100.00000   4.64158

48.   0.00000
       0.04000
       0.00000
       0.21000

       0.60000

49. 11.33900   24.78100   329.62736   8.11945   −1.65553

50.   ITEM 7 OUT OF RANGE   −30.00
                       ITEM 9 OUT OF RANGE   93.20
                       ITEM 13 OUT OF RANGE   −28.60

51.
```
ITEM NO.  5 IS NEGATIVE
ITEM NO. 10 IS NEGATIVE
ITEM NO. 11 IS NEGATIVE
ITEM NO. 17 IS NEGATIVE
ITEM NO. 20 IS NEGATIVE
```

52.

MEAN	EXPONENTIAL FORM
14.25	0.1424600E+02

53. CARD OUT OF SEQUENCE FOLLOWING NUMBER 151

54.
```
 B =    0.00423
 A =   27.57754
SYX =   47.71106
 R =    0.00164
```

55.

X	ALOG	SQRT
1.0	0.0000	1.0000
1.1	0.0953	1.0488
1.2	0.1823	1.0954
1.3	0.2624	1.1402
---	---	---
2.0	0.6931	1.4142

56.

MPH	1 MILE		2.5 MILES		5 MILES	
	MIN	SEC	MIN	SEC	MIN	SEC
45	1	20.0	3	20.0	6	40.0
46	1	18.3	3	15.7	6	31.3
47	1	16.6	3	11.5	6	23.0
48	1	15.0	3	7.5	6	15.0
65	0	55.4	2	18.5	4	36.9

57. Exact copy of your own source program.

58.
ALA.	6.65
ARIZ.	16.03
ARK.	25.30
CAL.	24.26

MASS.	25.11

59. As illustrated in the exercise.

60.   SUM = 270.35

61.
5	ALA.
15	ARIZ.
17	ARK.
48	CAL.

6	MASS.

62.
```
        64.20
        17.00
         0.00
        42.30
        ----
        19.00
```

63.   AVG. DEV. = 14.5020

64.
ITEMS		VALUES		MEAN	
1	2	19.00	0.04	9.520	
1	3	19.00	3.00	11.000	
1	4	19.00	5.21	12.105	
1	5	19.00	6.00	12.500	(36 lines of output)
---	---	---	---	---	
8	9	19.60	15.00	17.300	

65.   Y = 387062.47

66.

A	L
0.00	13
0.04	6
0.04	2
3.00	11

64.20	15

67.

EQUAL PAIRS
2 AND 6
3 AND 11
4 AND 16
13 AND 18

68.

5.21	−4.21	−40.60	14.60
47.30	28.60	28.30	6.00
0.00	27.50	−30.00	28.70
48.20	0.04	7.20	−4.30
20.60	2.45	21.20	15.00
6.00	9.38	−20.30	93.20
−3.20	9.21	19.60	5.70

69.

COLUMN SUMS

361.20	553.08	130.18	263.41	204.42

70. As illustrated in the exercise.

71. THETA

(DEGREES)	P1	P2	P3	P4	P5	P6
0	1.00000	1.00000	1.00000	1.00000	1.00000	1.00000
1	0.99985	0.99955	0.99909	0.99848	0.99772	0.99681
2	0.99940	0.99818	0.99635	0.99392	0.99089	0.98725
3	0.99863	0.99590	0.99180	0.98634	0.97955	0.97142
10	0.98481	0.95477	0.91057	0.85321	0.78400	0.70448

72. As illustrated in the exercise.

73. CHI-SQUARE = 4.50

74. As illustrated in the exercise.

75.

VARIABLES	R
1 AND 2	−0.26739
1 AND 3	0.29405
1 AND 4	0.03888
1 AND 5	0.38690
2 AND 3	−0.26359
2 AND 4	−0.19719
2 AND 5	−0.01763
3 AND 4	−0.06329
3 AND 5	−0.18886
4 AND 5	0.47273

76.

1.6667
8.0000
125.0000
15.0000
2.0000

77.

ALOG	SERIES	EXPONENT
0.405465	0.405465	9.0

(The exponent may vary, with computer precision)

78.

100.0000
4.0000

79. Test by trying various combinations of console switches.

80.

MORE THAN ONE NEGATIVE VALUE IN SET—
3
4
5
6
8
9

81. See Exercise 76.

82.

YEAR	INDEX
1	0.6503
2	3.1061
3	1.0000
4	1.8668
----	-------
10	−1.3217

83. Check result with Table 6, Chapter 3.

84.

MOVING AVERAGE — 20 ITEMS, PERIOD 12

13.2242
11.6408
13.0542
18.1542

23.3342

85.

12074 SECONDS

86.

12074 SECONDS

87.

3 HOURS
21 MINUTES
14 SECONDS

88.

	FORSYTH	BY MULTIPLICATION
10	0.3628787E+07	0.3628800E+07
20	0.2432900E+19	0.2432902E+19
30	0.2652528E+33	0.2652528E+33

89.

$M = -4$

90.

−1
0
1
2

91.

MEAN $= -13.195$

92.

MEAN $= 24.600$

93.

RADIANS	DEGREES	MINUTES	SECONDS
1	57	17	44.8
3	171	53	14.4
5	286	28	44.0
7	401	4	13.6
9	515	39	43.3

94.   HARMONIC MEAN = 0.1962

95.

A	L	
0.04	2	(first set)
0.04	6	
0.00	3	(second set)
0.00	8	
−40.60	10	(third set)
−4.21	3	
28.60	4	

96.

	A	B	R
ACTUAL VALUES	20.96639	−0.01197	0.00635
LOGARITHMS	2.81014	−0.13942	0.41404

97.

	BASE E	BASE 10
A	0.07292	−0.03167
B	0.30329	0.13172

PROJECTIONS— 19.3   26.1   35.4   47.9

98.   SUM OF SQUARES = 11220.9641
                  SQUARED SUM   = 61409.7961

99. Check precision with Table 6, Chapter 3, and Table 20, Chapter 10.

100.   1.5828   −2.7354

101.

P	Q	P AND Q	NOT (P AND Q)	NOT P	NOT Q	NOT P AND NOT Q	NOT P OR NOT Q
T	T	T	F	F	F	F	F
F	T	F	T	T	F	F	T
T	F	F	T	F	T	F	T
F	F	F	T	T	T	T	T

102. Test on invented data.

103.

	A	B	C	LS	RS
1	T	T		T	T
	T	F		T	T
	F	T		F	F
	F	F		F	F
2	T	T		T	T
	T	F		T	T
	F	T		F	F
	F	F		F	F
3	T	T		T	T
	T	F		T	T
	F	T		T	T
	F	F		F	F
4	T	T		T	T
	T	F		F	F
	F	T		F	F
	F	F		F	F
5	T	T	T	T	T
	T	T	F	F	F
	T	F	T	T	T
	F	T	T	T	T
	F	F	T	F	F
	F	T	F	T	T
	T	F	F	F	F
	F	F	F	F	F
6	T	T	T	T	T
	T	T	F	T	T
	T	F	T	F	F
	F	T	T	T	T
	F	F	T	T	T
	F	T	F	F	F
	T	F	F	F	F
	F	F	F	F	F

104.

	X	DEV	DEV**2
1	19.00	0.94	0.88
2	0.04	−18.02	324.72
3	3.00	−15.06	226.80
4	5.21	−12.85	165.12
20	20.60	2.54	6.45

(check with both FORMAT statements)

105.

	X	DEV	DEV**2
1	1900.00	94.00	8836.00
2	4.00	−1802.00	3247204.00
3	300.00	−1506.00	2268036.00
4	521.00	−1285.00	1651225.00
20	2060.00	254.00	64516.00

106.

	X	DEV	DEV**2
1	8836.00	94.00	8836.00
2	3247204.00	−1802.00	3247204.00
3	2268036.00	−1506.00	2268036.00
4	1651225.00	−1285.00	1651225.00
20	64516.00	254.00	64516.00

107.

JONES 2.30

SMITH 2.14

108.

BCV =	574.7435
WCV =	753.2284
F =	0.7630
D.F. =	3, 96

109.

	L.T. 0	16
0	L.T. 10	40
10	L.T. 20	14
20	L.T. 30	13
	G.E. 100	1
	TOTAL	100

110.

JAN	0.574
FEB	0.486
MAR	1.243
APR	0.944
MAY	0.831
JUN	1.564
JUL	1.513
AUG	1.502
SEP	0.894
OCT	0.775
NOV	0.652
DEC	1.022
YEAR	12.000

111. Test as suggested in the exercise.

112.

B	XI(1)	N(1)	XI(2)	N(2)	XI(3)	N(3)
1.0	NO ROOTS					
2.0	1.8955	4				
3.0	2.2788	2				
4.0	2.4745	3				
5.0	2.5957	4	4.9063	3		
6.0	2.6788	4	5.2258	3		
7.0	2.7395	4	5.4017	3		
8.0	2.7859	4	5.5210	2	7.9574	3
9.0	2.8226	4	5.6101	3	8.2610	3
10.0	2.8523	4	5.7689	3	8.4232	4

(N = number of iterations)

113.

N = 20   MEDIAN = 16.00
N = 25   MEDIAN = 15.00

114.

"THE" OCCURS   3   TIMES

115.

ANESTHETIC
BEGINNINGS
SURGICAL
TECHNIQUE

116.
$$A = \ \ 9.82955$$
$$B = -0.20930$$
$$C = -0.0011094$$

117. Exact area $= 8.57977$.

118. Check by inspection.

119. May be checked by inspecting Exercise 120 results.

120. Check by inspection of distribution and diagram.

appendix B

SUMMARY COMPARISON OF FORTRAN COMPILERS

The summary table that follows does not incorporate the detail available in the 25 individual tables that appear throughout the text. It is intended as a quick reference for major characteristics of various FORTRAN compiler programs.

The short title that appears for each compiler lists only the lowest number computer for which the compiler is available. Full identification of all computers and manufacturers appears in the compiler index following the Contents.

Descriptive notation used in the summary table is explained below, and the applicable text table containing detail is noted.

Column

1 *Statement continuation*—The number presented is maximum total lines for any statement, including the first.
   UL = unlimited
    C = limit stated as maximum number of separate characters
    ? = number not stated in manufacturer's manual
   NA = statement continuation not allowed

   See Table 1.

2 *Variable names*—The number presented is maximum total characters in the variable name. (In some cases, more characters may appear, but are ignored by the compiler.)
    ? = number not stated in manufacturer's manual

   See Table 2.

3 *Statement numbers*—The number presented is the maximum permissible statement number

   See Table 4.

Column

4   *Real range*—The number presented is the maximum permissible size of exponents (e.g., ± 38 represents $\#(10)^{\pm 38}$ or, in FORTRAN, $\#E \pm 38$. Note that in some instances the size of $\#$ is limited, for the maximum exponent value.)

? = range not stated in manufacturer's manual

See Table 6.

5   *Real single precision*—The number presented is the number of significant digits stored in single precision.

CC = determined by control card

? = precision not stated in manufacturer's manual

See Table 6.

6   *Real double precision*—The number presented is the number of significant digits stored in double precision.

? = Double precision available, but precision not stated in manufacturer's manual

NA = Double precision not available

See Table 20.

7   *Integer range*—The number presented is the maximum number of digits available for integer storage. More precise limits appear in Table 10. For example, where "7" appears below, the limit may be 9,999,999, 8,388,607, or 2,097,151, and so on.

REAL = all arithmetic done in real mode.

See Table 10.

8   *Double precision variables*

√ = available via explicit type declaration

CC = available via control cards

NA = not available

See Tables 20, 21.

9   *Complex variables*

√ = available via explicit type declaration

NA = not available

See Table 22.

Column

10   *Logical variables*
        √ = available via explicit type declaration
        NA = not available

See Table 23.

11   *Mixed expressions*—Refers specifically to combination of REAL and INTEGER modes in arithmetic expressions.
        √ = allowed (integers floated for the computation)
        ? = not stated in manufacturer's manual
        NA = not allowed (usually results in compilation error: "mixed mode")

See Table 10.

12   *Subscripts; form*
        USAS = matching U.S.A. Standard for FORTRAN IV; all forms of (integer) constant ∗ variable ± constant
        IE = any integer expression may appear as subscript
        AE = any arithmetic expression may appear as subscript
        LIM = limited; less flexibility than U.S.A. Standard for FORTRAN IV
        ? = subscript form not stated in manufacturer's manual

See Table 13.

13   *Subscripts; maximum dimensions*—The number presented is the maximum number of dimensions for any array.
        UL = unlimited
        ? = maximum not stated in manufacturer's manual

See Table 14.

14   *Input/output statement form*
        II = FORTRAN II form; generally PUNCH f, PRINT f, READ f, and specific tape statements
        IV = FORTRAN IV form; generally WRITE (u,f) and READ (u,f)
        II, IV = compiler accepts both forms
        U = unusual form of input/output statements

See Tables 3, 7.

Column

15   *Input/output unit control statements*—Usually BACKSPACE u, RE-
      WIND u, END FILE u (or ENDFILE u).
            √ = available
            NA = not available

See Table 8.

16   *Alphameric; literal transfer*
            √ = available (followed by appropriate character used to enclose
                the literal string)
            NA = not available

See Table 11.

17   *Alphameric; A Format*—The number presented is maximum field
      width (usually for REAL variable names).
            CC = field width depends on control cards
            ? = A Format available, but maximum field width not stated in
                manufacturer's manual
            NA = A Format not available

See Table 11.

18   *Printer carriage control*
            USAS = matching U.S.A. Standards for FORTRAN IV (blank =
                single space, 0 = double space, 1 = sheet eject or
                1–9 = skip to channels 1–9, + = suppress space)
            USAS+ = more control characters than U.S.A. Standard for
                FORTRAN IV
            LIM = fewer control characters than U.S.A. Standard for
                FORTRAN IV
            NA = no arrangement for printer carriage control

See Table 12.

19   *Scale factor*—Refers to "P" notation in FORMAT.
            √ = available
            NA = not available

See Table 24.

Column

20   *FORMAT as data array*—Refers to treatment of FORMAT statement as data read at execution time in "A" Format.

        √ = available

      NA = not available

                                                   See Table 25.

21   *FORTRAN-Supplied Functions*

          II = FORTRAN II form (usually, function names ending in F)

          IV = FORTRAN IV form

      II, IV = both forms acceptable to compiler

            ? = no functions listed in manufacturer's manual

                                           See Tables 5, 19.

22   *Adjustable dimensions*—Refers to permissibility of integer variables in subprogram DIMENSION statements (repeated as subprogram arguments).

        √ = available

      NA = not available

                                                 See Table 18.

23   *Labeled COMMON*

        √ = available

      NA = not available

                                                 See Table 18.

24   *CALL EXIT*—Refers to FORTRAN statement calling a subprogram that returns control to a supervisory or monitor program.

        √ = available

      NA = not available

                                                 See Table 9.

25   *Switch statements*—Refers to both "External" and "Internal" (including "imaginary") switches.

          II = FORTRAN II form (usually IF statements)

          IV = FORTRAN IV form (usually CALL statements)

      II, IV = Both forms available

          NA = no switch reference statements available

                                         See Tables 16, 17.

Column

26   *DATA Statement*
        √ = available
        NA = not available

See Table 25.

27   *Hollerith constant*—Refers to use of nH or literal transfer in DATA statement, and as arguments in CALL statements.
        √ = available
        NA = not available

See Table 25.

INDEX